"An exquisitely thoughtful book, always provocative, wise beyond words. Mr. Hayes has a lovely spirit and strong insights into the springs of personal power. My highest recommendation."

—**John Taylor Gatto**, former New York Teacher of the Year; author of *The Underground History of American Education*

"*The Rapture of Maturity* takes the reader on a wonderful intellectual journey through the author's own lived experiences as well as some timeless scholarly works on the mysteries of human existence. The book is a rich tapestry in which threads of insight are interwoven by the author into a fabric of wisdom, providing the reader with a comforting blanket of understanding regarding some of the more distressing aspects of being human.

"Charles Hayes does this by building insight upon insight, showing us that we can develop a heightened awareness of life's mental treasures by reflecting on, and engaging in, true learning about one's self and the world. This book will appeal to adults of all ages who are seeking a mature existence in an otherwise superficial world. Those who are in the second half of life and engaged in a review of life's meanings will find this both inspiring and comforting. Those who are nearing middle age and want to ensure that their second half of life is ripe with meaning will find this to be a valuable guide for directing their lives. And, those young people who see through the banality of a popular culture that is trying to cajole them into shortsighted lifestyles will take pause and consider the wisdom of the ages."

—**James Côté**, author of *Arrested Adulthood: The Changing Nature of Maturity and Identity*

PRAISE FOR *PORTALS IN A NORTHERN SKY*

"Reading *Portals* is like looking through a kaleidoscope in which break-neck adventure and science fiction occasionally reconfigure themselves into patterns of ancient wisdom—don't start unless you have enough time to finish it, because you won't be able to put it down."

—Mihaly Csikszentmihalyi, author of
Flow and *The Evolving Self*

"Charles Hayes, one of the great existential pathfinders of the modern age, has produced a masterpiece, a work of genius, in the form of *Portals in a Northern Sky*. This fascinating and exquisitely crafted story unfolds against a sweeping landscape of nature, history, and culture, and is woven together into a magnificent tapestry of insight and wisdom. Hayes takes the reader on an unforgettable journey that unveils lost secrets about the art of creative and meaningful living. *Portals in a Northern Sky* is the ultimate thinking person's novel, one that is certain to become a classic for future generations to enjoy and cherish. Absolutely essential reading."

—John F. Schumaker, author of *Wings of Illusion*
and *The Age of Insanity*

"A fascinating tale, well-told, that moves backward and forward in time. By themselves, the references to classic literature and philosophers make the book valuable at any price."

—Jack Roderick, author of *Crude Dreams: A Personal
History of Oil & Politics in Alaska*

"*Portals in a Northern Sky* is a delightfully different book, truly in a class by itself—among other things a science-fiction novel, a thriller, a meditation on fate, and a love letter to Alaska. Readable and rewarding on all counts."

—Walter Truett Anderson, author of *The Truth
About the Truth* and *All Connected Now*

THE RAPTURE
OF MATURITY

THE RAPTURE OF MATURITY

A Legacy of Lifelong Learning

CHARLES D. HAYES

Autodidactic Press

Library of Congress Catalog No. 2004104862

ISBN 0-9621979-4-7

Printed in the United States of America

Cover and interior design by Lightbourne, Inc.

10 9 8 7 6 5 4 3 2 1

First Edition

Autodidactic Press
P. O. Box 872749
Wasilla, AK 99687

www.autodidactic.com

Publisher's Cataloging-in-Publication
(Provided by Quality Books, Inc.)

Hayes, Charles D. (Charles Douglas)
  The rapture of maturity : a legacy of lifelong
learning / Charles D. Hayes.
    p. cm.
    Includes bibliographical references and index.
    LCCN 2004104862
    ISBN 09621979-4-7

  1. Self-culture. 2. Non-formal education--United
States. 3. Aging--Philosophy. 4. Culture--Philosophy.
5. Social change. I. Title

LC32.H39 2004   374
                   QBI33-2023

Dedicated to the memory of my grandparents,
Charles T. and **Pansy M. Enochs**

ACKNOWLEDGMENTS

The subject of this book has been on my mind for many years. In some cases, I've taken bits and pieces of past essays and newsletter articles that have continued to simmer in my imagination and have reworked them in an effort to get them right. It's a process that never ceases, and once in a while putting my thoughts into print allows me enough detachment to revisit a subject with new perspective. The contradictions in this work remain my property and my primary preoccupation.

I'm fortunate to have had the assistance of several people who have offered helpful advice and ongoing support. They are: Carolyn Acheson, Mike Chmielewski, James R. Fisher, Jr., Ronald Gross, Jack Roderick, Sonya Senkowsky, my sister Cheryl Wright, and my wife, Nancy. I'm also deeply indebted to many of the authors listed in this work. Shelley E. Taylor's *Positive Illusions* has remained on the front burner of my awareness since I first read it in 1989. In similar fashion, so have Ronald Gross' *Independent Scholar's Handbook*, Mihaly Csikszentmihalyi's *Flow*, Jared Diamond's *Guns, Germs and Steel*, Daniel C. Dennett's *Darwin's Dangerous Idea*, and Alan Watts' *Wisdom of Insecurity*.

Most of all, I'm grateful for the assistance of my editor, LuAnne Dowling, who has been bringing clarity to my rambling for nearly two decades.

CONTENTS

PREFACE

*The greatest discovery of any generation
is that a human being can alter his life
by altering his attitude.*
—William James

When thoughts of our own mortality begin to crop up with increasing frequency, it's time to pause and contemplate our legacy. We're reminded to ask ourselves what of value we intend to leave for posterity. After the tangibles of the estate are settled, what will our successors remember about us? Is there something we can do now that will generate a lasting, positive effect in the lives of our descendants?

We've witnessed a breathtaking acceleration in the pace of daily life during the past century. Appearances are deceiving, however. Unrelenting change may sometimes feel like progress, but it is often a threat to our best-laid plans. A painful case in point is the recent divorce of my granddaughter's parents, an episode that marks the first instance of this kind of separation in my family in five generations. I take little comfort in knowing that millions of others are confronted with similar situations. Relational matters are growing in complexity, and the rate of family disintegration continues to climb. Now, more than ever, the bonds between older and younger generations represent crucial connecting points for building a more promising future.

My grandparents were born near the turn of the twentieth century. World War I and the simultaneous flu pandemic left many of their contemporaries with a profound sense of disillusionment. Intellectuals of the period referred to theirs as the Lost Generation. In *A Farewell to Arms,* Ernest Hemingway wrote about the war as an experience in which glory, sacrifice, and sacredness were just words that had lost their meaning. And yet, my grandfather, himself a veteran of that war, was anything but lost. He and my grandmother left me with an intense appreciation for maturity as an attribute of adulthood. As a result, I feel a profound sense of connection with the values of an era that is gone forever. The time I spent with my grandparents was glorious, their sacrifices for our family were obvious, and the memories I hold are sacred indeed.

My grandfather was born in Ohio in 1889; my grandmother in Tennessee in 1904. They were Victorians, both in character and in aspiration. But to my granddaughter born in 1994, they represent a world so different from ours of today that they might as well have come from another planet.

The times in which we live contribute to shaping our values. In the 1950s, David Riesman's book *The Lonely Crowd* identified a tectonic shift in the nature of individual motivation. Riesman observed that people of the current generation were becoming increasingly "other-directed." That is, they were acting in response to the expectations of others, doing things because of what other people thought, as opposed to being "inner-directed" and doing things simply because they were the right things to do. The change was something philosopher Søren

Kierkegaard had predicted a century before: loss of the individual at the expense of mass-man. I recall at least one sociologist who maintained that the Victorians had lived their whole lives as a pose. But how does this view square with the idea that they were inner-directed? Long hours of reflection about my grandparents have led me to formulate an answer.

Every generation strikes a pose, but the nature of the motivation behind that pose can vary greatly. The character and disposition of my grandparents' era stand out in sharp contrast to the distinctive attributes of my parents' generation and to those of my own. Of course, there have always been individuals with exceptional sources of motivation, but my impression is that my grandparents represented the period before the great motivational shift described by Riesman. They belonged to the last generation of those who were largely inner-directed. Certainly they were concerned about what other people in their society thought of them, but that wasn't the criterion by which they made their everyday decisions. Rather, they made their choices solely on the basis of what they thought was the right thing to do—the opposite motivation from those who are other-directed.

My grandfather volunteered for service in World War I so that his brother could remain at home and work the family farm. As a working man with young children during the Great Depression, he sharpened his skill at thriftiness and was frugal to a fault for the rest of his life. He lived by deeply held principles, and if you spent enough time with him you could figure out what those were without need of an explanation. He and my grandmother accepted total responsibility for themselves and their family. They neither asked for nor expected help from anyone. Initiative was an inborn part of their psychological makeup. They didn't need to be lectured about self-reliance; it was a big part of who they were. They tended their own garden, canned their own food, and supplemented their mechanical needs with their own ingenuity. My grandfather paid his bills on time and in person. My grandmother was an extraordinarily resourceful homemaker and made many of the family's clothes. The two of them did these things without any regard, whatsoever, for what others thought of their actions. Admittedly, their generation committed its share of blunders, and many people suffered the ethnocentric prejudices of previous and subsequent generations, but my grandparents embodied an aspect of maturity that continues to outshine our present-day standards.

Today, on the surface at least, my granddaughter's generation seems to be consumed by peer pressure. If not dissuaded, she'll soon count among those who have internalized "shopping mall values" to such an extent that they feel incomplete without proper brand-name tags on their clothing. The absence of inner-directedness is frightening. Comparing such values to those of my grandparents makes me profoundly nostalgic about the concept of authenticity. I suspect this is because one of the most readily observable aspects of inner-directedness is earnestness. My grandparents' generation was wrong about many things in life, but their worldview was never pessimistic or sarcastic. To me and my siblings, they represented optimism, steadfastness, stability and, above all, sincerity. I believe my granddaughter's generation possesses a similar capacity for sincerity. Yet I fear that, if the peer pressure they endure does not lessen, they will be overtaken in the near future by a deep-seated sense of irony and a penchant for cynicism.

Unfortunately, not everyone is privileged to have fond memories of strong ties to individuals substantially older than themselves. Some people grow up not knowing their grandparents or an equivalent at all; some experience strained relationships at best. And, of course, the farther back we go in time, the less likely it is that a generation would even remember the earlier ones because life expectancy used to be so much shorter. Nonetheless, when these relationships do exist in a constructive way between young and old, whether related family members or not, they have the potential to seed future generations with some of the most worthwhile qualities of the past.

Like a comet in the night sky, a lasting inspiration from one generation offers a distant, succeeding generation something of genuine and enduring value. It creates an effervescent link from one century to another—an oblique but thoughtful message, from those the youth did not know and will not remember, passed on to a time the elders will never see.

Each new generation longs for what it grew up without, and each generation in decline longs for something it once admired but deems lost. Ensuring that every generation is capable of projecting vitality into future generations requires a willingness to reevaluate one's own values—it's the only way we can squeeze the last drop of meaning from our past experience. Change is always to be expected, yet there is something in our nature that at some point makes us want to push away from life's table and say, "Enough for me." If you hear people expressing relief that they won't be here when such and such happens in the future, it's a telltale sign of surrender.

My grandfather was fourteen when the Wright brothers first flew an airplane. By the time my granddaughter was born, our moon landings seemed like ancient history. When my grandparents first moved to Oklahoma from Tennessee, traffic on the road was so sparse that every time they met a car coming toward them, both drivers would automatically pull over, eager to discuss road conditions. Considering how strange these comparisons sound today, imagine how outlandish they will seem in 2189.

Today's literature for seniors offers repeated warnings about obtaining parental approval before giving advice to children. Without question, a strong relationship between children and their parents is vital for a healthy future, but I must leave that topic for others to write about. My focus here is on adults in the September of life and the fact that the relationship between grandparents and grandchildren has always been regarded as special. Some people joke that the two get along so well because they share a common enemy: the parents. Whatever truth exists in the humor of that observation, I imagine one of the main reasons is that grandparents and grandchildren both share a time orientation more appreciative of the present than that of their career-burdened parents, consumed with past debts and planning ahead. If we can successfully distinguish the traits we admired so much in our elders and build them into the repertoire of our own behavior, we will need no one's permission to pass on a legacy given to us long ago by people whose lives were most worthy of a lasting and cherished remembrance.

Any generation can be lost if the greatest attributes and aspirations of its members are not passed on. From as far back in time as I can remember, I dreaded the inevitable death of my grandparents. And now, in memory, they clearly seem to have lived in another time, in a far away place. Change has erased most of the evidence that they ever lived. All that's left is my enduring sense of regret over their absence and my determination to emulate the values they stood for. If the love, courage, imagination, and special wisdom of their generation are misplaced, they will indeed have been a Lost Generation, and that would be a tragedy. What the words, *glory, sacrifice,* and *sacredness* will mean in the twenty-second century I can't predict, but now that my grandparents are gone and I am a grandparent myself, I can see glaring differences between generations that must be addressed by mature individuals.

Whether you are a parent, grandparent, or fill the role of a surrogate, *The Rapture of Maturity* is about each and every one of us striving to make the most of our lives. The degree of maturity we achieve will affirm the value of the effort we have made to get there. In writing this book, I'm hopeful that I might be able to pass on something from my grandparents to my granddaughter's grandchildren, with or without need of explanation. I further hope that, after reading this book, you will feel motivated to do the same for the young people in your life and the generations that follow.

INTRODUCTION

The universe is change;
life is what thinking makes of it.
—Marcus Aurelius

Amerian mythologist Joseph Campbell once said that what most people are searching for is the "rapture of being alive." The idea may not apply to everyone everywhere, but exploration of it may shed more light on improving quality of life than all of the advice offered during the second half of the twentieth century by America's army of self-help gurus. Rapture is often defined as being in a state of ecstasy, or of being carried away in body and/or spirit with a sense of joy. It's portrayed as a rare experience that we don't very often talk about. Indeed, we learn as children that we must forsake ecstasy in favor of behavior more acceptable to our parents and community.[1] We create selves who conform at the expense of expressing what we really feel. So, to say that adults can expect to experience rapture may seem far-fetched, but that doesn't make the goal any less desirable. Who can deny the ecstasy of ecstasy? By comparison, the pursuit of happiness seems tame if not trivial.

Examples abound in the world's great literature describing the ecstasy of discovery, of sensual pleasure, and of sublime mystical experience. Firsthand accounts from soldiers in battle tell us of their heightened feelings of being alive when their lives were in imminent danger. In times of relative peace, we may observe a resurgence in popularity of high-risk activities, from skydiving and bungee jumping to snow boarding, among individuals seeking that same feeling. Such youthful, thrill-seeking behavior seems more like an escape than a path to bliss, however, in an era of global conflict, economic insecurity, environmental degradation, and human starvation.[2] In contrast, the rapture of maturity emerges from reflection and welcomes new insight about these matters.

After more than two decades of extensive self-education, I have become increasingly conscious that writers can spend years and hundreds of thousands of words trying to solve the same existential problems that prompted them to start writing in the first place. In that regard I am no exception. My quest has been to show that the quality of our existence depends upon learning. By learning I mean, not the rote memorization of facts, but sincere efforts aimed at better understanding the very nature of knowledge and the tenuous, cultural construction of the things we call reality. I've come to the conclusion that rapture and maturity are reciprocal products of authenticity, and that authenticity involves living your life as if you are really interested in it.

Clearly there are many activities in life, apart from intellectual endeavors, that are extraordinarily meaningful. Even so, regardless of who you are and where your interests lie, nothing substitutes for thinking, and no one is exempt from the need to do so. Excitement from dangerous activity, though exhilarating, is not an effective substitute for the mental effort necessary to reach emotional and intellectual maturity. Thrill-seeking activities are not always the heroic, death-defying feats they appear to be. Sometimes these acts mask intellectual fears of annihilation. It's often easier to take chances than to contemplate nothingness.

Hackneyed though it may sound, the fear of death ultimately amounts to a fear of life and a sense of insignificance. In tending to people on their deathbeds, Rabbi Harold S. Kushner has said that the individuals who have the most trouble with death are the ones who felt they had never really lived.[3] They dread insignificance.[4] Similarly, we observe that people on the verge of success often sabotage their own efforts, but we seldom recognize that one of the reasons they do this is to avoid making their existential dilemma of existence even greater than it already is: if they are indeed able to experience a rapturous existence, then their deep-seated fear of death becomes magnified and their loss all the greater.[5]

My definition of rapture, for the purpose of this book, is similar to the idea of being swept up in a great sense of joy, but not as a one-time experience. Rapture may come in a multitude of subtle but insightful flashes of realization that life is indeed worth living, coupled with the inspiration that, given a choice, we would trade places with no one on this planet. The rewards we gain from intellectual efforts are the highest our species can reap. What holds us back is our culture.

When I use the term "intellectual," I don't have in mind groups of elites whose need to be above it all takes the form of pretentiousness designed to hide a fear of being understood.[6] In my view, an intellectual is someone who thinks deeply about matters that deserve such attention. Unfortunately, American popular culture is vengefully anti-intellectual. You don't have to watch late-night television comedians interviewing people on the street to know that many of our fellow Americans suffer arrested intellectual development, which, in the shadow of our great wealth, is a travesty. Millions of people forgo the pursuit of knowledge, settling instead for mindless entertainment to offset the pain of an unfulfilling life. This happens in spite of the fact that we know lifelong learning represents a literal fountain of youth. People with a thirst for knowledge live longer and better lives. Plain old everyday experience offers countless clues to validate that learning adds quality to our lives. Doesn't everything that ceases to grow begin to die? Brains atrophy, just as muscles do when they are underutilized.

Learning as a principal elixir of life is hardly a secret to those whose quest for understanding is never satiated. People who spend their lives learning vitalize themselves and those with whom they associate. On the one hand, people who seem interested in everyone and everything going on around them radiate with enthusiasm. On the other hand, whether rich or poor, those whose thirst for knowledge has never fully developed have little difficulty projecting boredom and despair at any age. Ralph Waldo Emerson once said, "Intellect annuls fate." If he was right, and I think the evidence clearly suggests he was, then contemplation is a path to maturity and authenticity. This mode of rapture is available only to those who reach for it.

So, rapture in the simplest sense amounts to the sheer intellectual joy of being alive and the fleeting moments when one appreciates the feeling as such. Intellectual vigor gives range to experiences that enable a person to enjoy many more occasions of value, simply because depth and breadth provide more opportunities for experiencing quality. Just as an excellent swimmer can find more pleasure in a bottomless pool than in a shallow one, all of us can garner more from life when our understanding represents a deep reservoir of knowledge.

I believe that understanding the dynamics of maturity offers us a last chance as individuals to live a life that really matters. Of course, this admits to varying degrees of experience. Few people will say their lives haven't mattered, regardless of the lives they've lived. And yet, when you read this book, I promise you will gain a better appreciation of the difference between what matters and what *really matters.* Marcus Aurelius' assertion that "life is what thinking makes of it" is worth repeating often to ourselves. If we believe that what we think can affect the quality of our lives, it is by definition true; if not, it is by design false. My reading of two thousand years of philosophical debate about what really matters in this life can be stated simply: What matters to us matters because it matters, and that's quite enough reason to care about such things.

Our brains have built-in pleasure centers, and these are activated by three primary stimuli: food, sex, and learning. Those of us in the developed world have enough riches to experience food and sex as aesthetic gratification. But too many underrate our most powerful pleasure: learning. This is a great irony in the problem of human inequality. Untold millions of people on earth starve to death each century. Only 20 percent of our species receive enough food during childhood to reach normal physical maturity without any kind of stunted development. For billions of people, sex and reproduction are part of a risky gamble to ensure their very survival.

If learning were a priority, the global situation would surely be different.

All living things born into this world experience a life cycle, but not all creatures reach maturity. Some creatures die in infancy, plucked up as food by larger species. Some life forms are destined by their genetics to behave without a will of their own. Only humans contemplate their own fate and worry over their own deaths and the personal legacies they will leave behind. The final stage of human development, I believe, includes the capacity for a sense of rapture. Such transcendence comes about when our desire to better understand the world helps to make it a better place for those who live on after us.

The endorphin rush of learning has sent our kind into outer space, to the depths of the ocean, and into the strands of our DNA, and yet millions upon millions of well-fed, robust people live their lives in varying states of arrested intellectual development. The goal of this book is to show that the answers to human inequality, the misrelating among people and cultures that leads to conflict and war, and the existential angst of frustrated individuals in the developed world all depend upon our pursuit of the rapture of maturity.

Apart from offering appropriate citations for source material, I have tried to use endnotes sparingly, but in some cases I have included them only to give a more complete explanation. Chapter One presents what I've characterized as properties of life. It offers opportunities to reexamine those avenues of life most of us think we truly understand but don't. Chapter Two is a cursory examination of the existential angst of the human condition with hopeful insights about coping and displacing inescapable anxiety. Chapter Three advocates a quest for knowledge, advice for teachers, an examination of education as understanding, and a discussion of anti-intellectualism—a theme which, along with wisdom and maturity, appears repeatedly throughout this work. Chapter Four revisits many of these ideas within the contexts of maturity, discovering what really matters in life, and how to leave the world a better place than we found it.

This book is the result of more than 25 years of voracious self-study and more than 60 years of lived experience. I have attempted to make it the shortest possible explanation of matters that I view as being critical to quality of life. The only reason I've been able to say these things in so few pages is that I've been thinking about them for a long, long time—so long that I trust they will matter as much to you as they do to me.

Chapter One

PROPERTIES OF LIFE

*The value of life does not lie in the number
of years but in the use you make of them.*
—Montaigne

Only one century ago, life expectancy in the developed world was little more than 46 years. Today we're living nearly twice as long. But what are we doing with those extra years? What do they teach us? Do we gravitate toward wisdom? Do we pass on what we've learned to our progeny? Does the knowledge gleaned from the added years help us improve our relationships with members of our family, our friends, and our fellow citizens of the world, or do we become closed-minded and self-absorbed, whittling away our time and dreading the inevitability of life's end?

My grandfather was born in 1889. He died in 1981 at the age of 92. During the last 25 years of his life, whenever he spoke about any event in the distant future, he would preface it by subtly suggesting that he might not be here when it happened. At the time I found his comments aggravating and unnecessarily pessimistic. But today, past 60, I understand why he said what he did. He had discovered the subjective truth of his own mortality. The idea that life is finite was no longer an abstraction. I haven't yet figured out if this tendency to hedge one's bet on a limited future is a way to avoid the embarrassment of having made plans one can't keep or whether it is just a way to remind oneself that time is short.

Most of us have spent the first half of our lives denying the inevitability of our own death, but something about turning 50 enables us to penetrate this barricade of self-deception just enough to stay dimly aware that the end of life is forthcoming. For those of us fortunate enough to have lived this long and remain in reasonably good health, I believe this period is the premium apportionment of life. This is a time when we can separate the wheat of wisdom from the chaff of experience. Let me propose an approach.

In many applications of computer software we are offered a pull-down menu with *properties* listed among the options. Open the properties icon and you will find underlying specifics relative to the subject at hand. The following headings in this chapter are subjects I have characterized as *properties of life*. My treatment of each of these properties is not intended to be exhaustive—only to present some underlying specifics relative to experiencing greater insight. The list is woefully incomplete and may seem arbitrary in content and order, but my hope is that you will use it to begin exploring the ways these properties have influenced your own life.

TIME

Isn't it amusing how those of us in the developed nations of the world have become so comfortable with using big numbers? We think nothing of mentioning a million here, a billion there. Mere hundreds of thousands are no big deal. But then, when you consider that human beings live only some thirty thousand days, give or take a few hundred, numbers begin to take on an entirely different perspective—at least, with respect to time. Our lives don't even amount to a million hours.

Since the emergence of Einstein's theory of relativity, scientists have told us that time and space are interchangeable and that gravity slows time. Geologists tell us there was once a much taller mountain range where the Rocky Mountains are now, that has been worn away over eons by the wind. The only thing you and I might really know about time is that, as the saying goes, it keeps everything from happening at once. But, if gravity slows time, can we even be sure we know that much? Throughout written history some very thoughtful philosophers have suggested, half in jest and half seriously, that time is circular, that everything that happens will happen again in an infinite stream of endless, seamless transactions. Stranger still is the inference from relativity theory that the past, present, and future exist simultaneously. We may sense moments in life when consciousness itself seems as if it might be a peculiar manifestation of time.

As children growing up, we assimilate the notion that time is a commodity. Time, we're told, is something we have that can be given, taken, or stolen from us, borrowed, squandered, killed, or set aside. Yet, on another plane, we perceive of time as movement that has a clearly discernible trajectory. We learn to think of time as a valuable but limited resource and eventually adopt the phrase "time is money" (even if we resent the idea). Time becomes a criterion for a series of investment decisions: how will we invest our time and what will be the payoff?

Strong interests and absorption in interesting activities make time seem to pass quickly. Indeed, we experience being truly focused as being lost in time. Though we may complain about being pressed for time, time pressures often tend to increase our personal happiness. When we are bored, or when we're forced to do something or be somewhere we would rather not, time seems to slow down. For years I worked a rotating week-on, week-off schedule for an oil company in the Arctic. The work itself was interesting enough, but the location was as desolate as the surface of the moon. When the airplane landed there each week, I felt as if we had entered a time warp where everything occurred in slow motion. When we returned to the city the following week, time seemed to switch to fast-forward again.

Clock time becomes increasingly important with technological progress. The clock asserts cultural pressure on us, commanding where, how, and when we will spend our time, when to stop, when to go, when to sleep, and when to work and play. In a matter of generations, we have moved from the hourglass to nanoseconds, from a time in which solitude in the absence of others dominated individual reality to times in which the front pages of our awareness are under assault by all sorts of media during most of our waking hours. Oddly enough, technological progress simultaneously reduces our leisure time while it enables us to do things faster. Worse, "busyness" increasingly takes on the appearance of virtue, even if the activity we are engaged in is itself absurd.

More than being a measure of one's lifespan, time sets the tone, tenor, and timbre of our existence. The pressure it brings to bear on our lives is alternately joyful and excruciating. In childhood, time seems to pass very slowly, at least in comparison to our experience as adults. A sense of urgency slows our perception of time. Wait for the pot to boil, and time stands still. When we're in it, childhood seems like a long, never-ending tunnel of experience, where the self that is "I" is always the same. Then, when we enter middle age, the years begin to pass by like telephone poles seen through the window of a fast-moving train. We may perceive ourselves as killing time, but ultimately we realize that it kills us. At this point, time becomes more valuable than money. This recognition can momentarily flood us with panic, with an overwhelming feeling that we need to stand up and pull the stop cord. Suddenly we must get a grip on the thing we call time before the trip is over, although we have yet to figure out where we really want to go.

Time is rich with cultural wisdom, but the very nature of wisdom has a fleeting quality, seeming available to us one moment and gone the next. The experiences of our ancestors and of the countless generations who preceded us have been recorded in literature, in texts about philosophy and psychology, and in a whole genre of life-stage theories by people interested in the aging process. Each generation, though, stumbles into new chapters of life with a sense of shock, as if they are discovering them for the first time for the whole of the human race. We make precious little use of the experiences of others except in hindsight comparison.

Ideas about values and community move through time with a metronomic tempo that makes the past appear far simpler than it was and the present far more complicated than it really is. In our effort to understand the nature of time, we find it to be both enduring and baffling. British philosopher Bryan Magee puts it this way: "Near the heart of the mystery of the world must be something to do with the nature of time. Whatever the truth about time may be, time cannot be what it seems."[7]

We perceive of eternity as endless time, but time itself is absent from the very notion of eternity. The character of eternity seems to be simply that eternity *is*. We perceive that our clocks and watches measure time, but this may be merely an illusion perpetrated by our brains. Life measures time, and perhaps it's not too far-fetched to think of ourselves as units of time. Eternity *is* as we *are*. Beyond that, little about time seems certain.

PLACE

The notion of place is often interchanged metaphorically with the concept of time, as when the future looms ahead, for example, or when a special place like heaven or utopia is said to be just beyond the horizon. Like time, the property of place—specifically the place where we are born and where we grow up—exerts tremendous pressure upon shaping our lives. Our time spent as children tends to warp our spatial perception of place. If, after many years, you revisit the places where you spent your childhood, everything typically looks smaller than you remember it.

Just as large bodies in space increase gravity and warp time, so do large bodies of culture shape our perceptions about time and place. One can plot a north-south, east-west grid on our planet and make a fairly accurate guess as to the kind of life people will have, based on where in the world they are born and where they continue to live.

Unfortunately, these same coordinates can also tell us a great deal about what an area's residents are likely to think, as worldviews tend to congeal in geographical clusters.[8]

We tend to carry with us the imprint of the place of our youth for the whole of our lives. Our geographical history is almost a physical part of us. Geography reveals communities of people bonded together by race, creed, religion, belief, worldview, and a sharing of values that compel them to speak their language with similar accents, to dress alike and to eat the same foods. In place resides the culture that we internalize so deeply at an early age that before long the way we see the world appears to us as the only way it could be.

Indeed, who we are, in large part, depends upon where we are. Self-evident as this may be, when we observe strangers from afar who appear very different from us, we fail to temper our opinions with the knowledge that we look just as alien to them. Instead, we choose to think of them as strange and of ourselves as normal.

The property of place can take us to the brink of understanding about our identity and to ultimate questions about purpose. When we explore our geographical location in space, we are reintroduced to time, since time and space are interchangeable. The result is that we become referentially lost in space. On the earth we can plot precise coordinates of latitude and longitude; we can pinpoint our location as so many miles north, south, east and west of this place or that. And yet, when we move beyond our sun, which is but a mediocre star in a pedestrian galaxy, our notions of direction become meaningless. When we are truly honest with ourselves, in terms of place, we become de-centered in time and our sense of self-importance evaporates into the mystery of deep space.

CHANGE

Change is a property of both time and place. Change is written into the very code of existence. Change is the god of time, the master of place. Change is the signature of life, writ deeply into the marrow of what we humans comprehend as meaning. Change inhabits the seasons, punctuated as they are by birth, growth, maturity, resignation, death, and renewal. Change is seed, youth, and maturity turned to rot, turned yet again to seed. Change makes life what it is, even as we simultaneously opt for an illusion of stability in which to live our everyday lives. Indeed, what we perceive as the grim reaper is merely the longest shadow cast through time by the properties of change.

Generation after generation of human beings have lived out their whole lives believing change to be the exception, failing to understand that it is instead the rule. The very nature of our individual temperaments rests on how our expectations meet with reality. Maturity properly understood and achieved equals realistic expectations—the more experience we have, the more realistic our expectations should be. A spoiled brat throws a fit when things don't go his or her way, but, if the nature of change remains a mystery to us as adults, our way of making sense of the world will always be defective in a very fundamental way. Our expectations will always be skewed, leading to anxiety, despair, and bouts of anger that make our lives far more miserable than they need to be. At times it will even seem that inanimate objects have it in for us. In spite of the fact that we know better intellectually, we will act as if the door that hits us when we run into it needs to be hit back.

Understanding change as an essential property of life is itself fundamental to moving with the flow of life instead of against it. Taking such a view does not preclude having the nerve to go against the grain or to wage an upstream battle for a just cause. Going with the flow of life means developing an orientation that recognizes what things we have control over and those that we don't. For change to be understood, it must always be expected. Acknowledging this does not imply that we must abandon our basic human need for order. Indeed, there is a temporal measure of order to be found within the very dynamics of change, and maturity is not possible without recognition of it. When we utilize our powers of observation in advanced capacity, we detect strands of order in areas where nothing but chaos appeared before.

Alan Watts left us this advice about change: "The only way to make sense out of change is to plunge into it, move with it, and join the dance."[9] Another way we learn about the character of change is found in our next property: regret.

REGRET

Regret is a property of time, place, change and the human condition. It is a built-in component of learning life's most important lessons, although we habitually relegate regret to those dark places beneath consciousness. The most unfortunate thing about regret is that we rarely use it as wisely as we could.[10]

As I grow older, one of the things I've become increasingly sensitive to is how often bad memories creep into my conscious awareness. In reality these are memories I would like to change, things I'd like to fix and put right. They may not be dramatic events or seem very important to my life's trajectory, but they are like judgments on the test of life, standing out as wrong answers. For example, I recall living in a boarding house for a few months in my early twenties. In the room next to mine was an old man in his eighties who often asked me to have dinner with him. Most of the time I was in too much of a hurry and declined. When I did accept his invitation, I ate quickly and never stayed very long. The recurring memory I have today sees through that old man's screen door to the table always set with an extra plate in case he might have company for dinner. Today I understand that he was lonely. Back then I didn't have the time or the patience to notice. Still, I must have known more than I realized or I would not have developed a desire to go back into the past and fill the place at his table.

The old man has been dead for years, now. Why would something like this matter to me today? Think about how many harsh things you've said to others that you wish you could take back. How many times were you rude, cruel, or simply insensitive, when it would now make a better recollection if it could be undone and put right? All of us have such moments lodged in our memories. Some are simple wrongs that long to be righted; some are so deep they will never resurface; some are events that we can never fully forget. One of the things I regret most today is having honored the nursing home administrator's wishes not to allow my grandmother to go back home for visits after she had been admitted. It may have been the easiest and most convenient option for the nursing home staff, but it was not the right thing to do. Had I listened to my conscience at the time, I wouldn't have gone along with it. Reflecting on this kind of unfinished business within our own minds prepares us for similar decisions in the future.

From time to time I hear adults reminiscing about their lives, and saying they would not do one thing differently if they had their lives to live over. I've often wondered what it would take for such individuals to bridge the gap, take full advantage of their experience, and recognize the countless opportunities that were blithely or stubbornly overlooked. But I'm also aware that the subtlety and profundity of this kind of question catches most people off-guard. The self-centeredness of their replies reveals more about their own lack of reflection than it does about their past regrets.

In her book *Regret: The Persistence of the Possible*, Janet Landman tells us that "Regret properly understood is the past alive in the present."[11] Indeed, I view regret as an inductive avenue into intellectual and emotional conundrums of unfinished business, offering genuine opportunities for learning through experience.[12] In other words, regret acknowledged and used creatively can be a method of improving our relationships in the future as a result of having better understood our failures in the past. In this way the property of regret can be turned into an aspiration for a better future.[13] Landman says, "[A]s long as there's regret, there's hope."[14]

Time and the biology of aging seem to push us toward insight. Perhaps the ability to reap wisdom from experience is an evolutionary mechanism intended to bolster the success of the generations who will outlive us. Surely the genes we have already passed on will fare better if we can contribute to the recipients some wisdom about living.

Viewed in this way, regret becomes a device through which we can learn deeply from our experience and pass to others the value of recognizing opportunities for creating better memories for themselves. We can do this armed with the wisdom that the present still provides opportunities to get it right the first time. We can convey this wisdom not by lecturing others about what they should do but by explaining our own actions as they occur. In other words, we can set an example by living as if we really care about what happens in the future.

LOVE AND PASSION

From the ancient Greeks to Shakespeare, from Lord Byron to Colette, and from tens of thousands of lesser-known writers to the smallest of valentines, the property of love has preoccupied our species for centuries. From epic romantic tragedies to simple acts of kindness toward neighbors, the dynamic of love fascinates us and binds us. Of all the properties of life, love surely wins the contest for being the most confusing.

The more we study love, the less we are sure we understand it. Novelist Milan Kundera attaches love to the property of time and has written that "love is the glorification of the present."[15] The implication is, no love, no life. Love changes meaning with respect to time and place and is perhaps the most prominent feature of regret—so much so that one can't focus on either for very long without thinking of the other.

Love as a property of life is bound to the concept of passion, not only in the context of romance but also as passion for life. Passion is a mysterious feature of existence. Some of us seem to have an excess of passion; some of us too little. Passion can't be given to us; we have it or we don't. Passion is best described metaphorically: it's the fire in the belly, the buzz in the bee, the rage of the storm, the bark in the dog. At times, passion seems to be the very essence of ourselves as individuals, and sometimes it seems more like an internal flame that waxes and wanes. A life devoid of passion is a life lived at room temperature. Passion misperceived becomes a destroyer of human relations. Passion misapplied is often called hatred.

FEAR AND HATRED

Time and place have a great deal to do with the objects of our fear as we grow up. If our fears are great enough, learning to hate is likely to follow. And, as with the property of love, regret will play a leading role in our hatred, regardless of whether we are the haters or the hated. Indeed, a significant portion of the literature our culture deems valuable derives from the premise that there is often a very fine line between the properties of love and hate, and that fear works to both ends. Often it is misperceptions about the nature of change that fuel our fear and hatred from the start.

In most cultures (and America is certainly no exception) fear becomes a political property to be used as an emotional prod. The more unreflective the group, the more effectively fear works, and the more often it is used. Nothing feeds fear and hatred like misperception and ignorance about the intentions of others, and yet common knowledge that such is the case seems to be of little value in moving beyond our misunderstandings with regard to others. Eric Hoffer put it this way: "Hatred is the most accessible and comprehensive of all unifying agents."[16]

Recognizing this, those who take time to be more reflective are less likely to react on impulse. They can work through their fears with reason and evaluate which ones are legitimate.[17]

Franklin Roosevelt asserted during World War II that "we have nothing to fear but fear itself." This statement is often quoted as an important feature of wartime, but it's equally applicable to everyday life. There is a dark irony in the realization that hatred is a unifying agent precisely because fear is often a misappropriated property to begin with. Learning to fear seems to be a hardwired animal instinct, just as getting sick from eating a particular food can make us avoid it for a lifetime. Moreover, there is something about spiders, snakes, and darkness that gives all primates the jitters. Not long ago, I was walking on a dirt road near a forest when the sudden hoof beats of a horse became louder and louder, prompting me to wheel around as if I were under attack. The sound had caused me to react instinctively, long before I figured out the source of the noise. I can only imagine how many thousands of people throughout history perceived hoof beats as the last sound they would ever hear, for in the next instant they sustained the shock of an assault by spear or sword. The visceral nature of the fear I felt bore universal qualities. It's only one step from that kind of fear to hatred.

The most unfortunate aspect of this very effective hardwired learning is that we overdo it. Most people have irrational fears that are totally out of sync with the likelihood that feared outcomes might occur. I hate to fly in commercial aircraft, even though I know intellectually that it's safer than driving a car. In his book *The Culture of Fear*, Barry Glassner shows in great detail why we are habitually so afraid

of the wrong things. We must learn to catch ourselves in the act. The unifying agency of hatred is too
often based on irrational and absurd assumptions
about "others," which makes it a tragic characteristic of human relations.

TRAGEDY

For centuries our species has left a clear record
of fascination with tragedy. We celebrate it in
books, plays, and movies. Although the plots vary,
the overarching theme of tragedy and our reaction
to it is still one of our major preoccupations. In her
book *Evil in Modern Thought*, Susan Neiman writes,
"Tragedy is about the ways that virtue and happiness fail to rhyme, for the want, or the excess, of
some inconsiderable piece of the world which happens to be the only thing that mattered."[18] To
appreciate why the nature of change is so often
misunderstood, we need only consider how many
of the dramas in our history are predicated on the
occurrence of the unexpected.

It's not the unexpected aspect of tragedy that fascinates me, however; it's the expected. In the
Western world we grow up with a sense of reality
shaped by an appreciation for drama, still based in
large part upon Aristotle's description of what a well-
written tragedy should consist of. His scheme for
tragedy was to portray highborn or larger-than-life
individuals engaged in plots involving complex relationships, heroics, betrayal, and catharsis.[19] Such
works of art are emotionally charged concoctions of
imagination, and they are egocentric in a commu-
nicative sense because these are stories we can
relate to personally, even if only in fantasy. We aspire
to heroics in love and war, appreciating the drama

that makes our lives seem to be of center-stage importance in the world. Over the centuries a democratizing effect has emerged in literature in that ordinary people have become the main characters; a wonderful contemporary example is Briony in Ian McEwan's *Atonement*. But for more than two decades I've been perplexed by the fact that the other kind of tragedy—the non-dramatic example of death by starvation that plays out daily around the planet—escapes our attention. I'm well aware that it may take me another twenty years to fully comprehend the implication, but I believe very strongly that somewhere in this incongruity is an insightful key to bettering human relations on a global scale. Moreover, I trust that it will indeed be a tragedy if we don't figure it out.

Some events in this world are so tragic that it's difficult to ever fully accept that they really took place. In such cases as Auschwitz, Buchenwald, Dachau, Mauthausen, and Treblinka, tragedy is a woefully inadequate descriptor.[20] Time does have healing properties, although the pain may never be fully alleviated, only numbed or anesthetized. There seem to be no satisfying answers as to why tragic things happen to some and not to others. Chance, change, and luck are downplayed as something to be associated with gaming, but change and chance play major roles in our lives.[21]

Humans have a bias for self-deception. We often take credit for accomplishments resulting from sheer good fortune. We like to see ourselves as individuals who would have risen to our particular levels of accomplishment in life, regardless of how different our pasts might have been. But to think that we could have been as successful as we are had we been born in the slums of Bangladesh is beyond absurd. An inherent arrogance plays to our worst human instincts. We may call it a tragedy when the child of neglectful parents is found starving in America, where such things ought not to happen, but we're unwilling to take into account the millions of other children who are starving to death around the world. Such a stance implies that tragedy has limits. Pondering this enigma, I'm haunted by the perceptive question Daniel C. Dennett asks each of us about the character of global poverty: "Would you settle docilely for a life of meaningless poverty, knowing what you know today about the world?"[22] I then have a follow-up question: If you were to die of starvation in spite of such knowledge, would that be a tragedy, or should we reserve the label for failed relationships and unavoidable catastrophe, as is our tradition in the arts?

Tragedy deconstructed offers us insightful access to the subjective character of our individual selves and enhances our ability to understand others. In the final analysis, however, there may be no occasion more tragic for human beings than simply failing to mature, failing to reach a point where what we are able to give back to society is equal to or greater than the tax of our existence. Save genocide, what greater tragedy could there be for a person than to have had a chance to live a life that really mattered but not to have seized the opportunity and taken advantage of it—of having been a person who aged but did not, in fact, mature? To borrow an image from Nietzsche, what greater misery is imaginable than living a life that would not be worth living for a second time? Could there be a greater concept of waste than a chance to live not taken? What would those whose lives were taken needlessly in their youth say to those of us who fail to live our lives to the fullest? In comparison to inanimate objects, all life is rapture.

MEMORY

Memory represents the mental attribute with which we attempt to still time and place, and to squeeze and force change into a context that favors our individual life circumstances. It's where we draw on the capacity to learn from our experiences involving love, regret, and hatred, and where we develop a perspective and attitude toward tragedy. We don't have to study memory to know that it has both a short-term and a long-term character or to know from many years of lived experience that, save drama, we have to really care about things to move them into long-term memory. Simply put, memory is the database of our raw experience. Like any database, it responds to queries in direct correspondence to the care and structure with which it has been created. Memory is also egocentric. Beneath consciousness resides a very nearly autonomous editor who requires little encouragement to alter files in favor of recollection more aesthetically pleasing to our egos.

As we age, memory increasingly becomes a major reference point for making judgments and a refuge for hiding from their consequences. Nowhere is the call for living your life as if you are really interested in it more important than in etching experience into memory. Indeed, in a very real sense, we are our own historians, and memories are our archives. Memories, however, occur in the present while creating an illusion of visiting the past. Alan Watts warned about the misuse of memory. In *The Wisdom of Insecurity,* he wrote, "The power of memories and expectations is such that for most human beings the past and the future are not *as* real, but *more* real than the present. The present cannot be lived happily unless the past has been 'cleared up' and the future is bright with promise."[23] This brings us to the properties of imagination and courage.

IMAGINATION AND COURAGE

Imagination is a mysterious mediator that operates, at least in part, somewhere between intellect and our sensory apparatus. It resides deeply and moves freely among the labyrinths of internalized metaphors with which we apprehend and thus comprehend the world. Striving to meet experience with meaningful response, imagination appears to exist of its own volition, and yet the experience of our species' most creative members suggest that imagination works best when its services are expected. We apply our imaginations to those things we truly care about. Necessity as the mother of invention rings true. Albert Einstein deemed imagination more important than knowledge, something to which his work attests. If knowledge were represented by a nail, imagination would be the hammer that puts it to use.

Courage is an attribute we apply to the individual, even though the process of defining courage is a socially collective effort. We deem those things courageous which others are likely to agree are courageous. It should not be lost on us that imagination and courage often represent a hand-in-glove response to a particular problem or situation. We often act imaginatively in perilous situations. Courage seems to be an article of character taken to a higher level, as if it is character's response to stress.

When you begin to think of imagination and courage as being closely related, the merger of the two takes the guise of a life force, part of our emotional stance toward living. When we think of a person who is both imaginative and courageous, for example, we are likely to have vivid ideas not only about how that person would act in times of crisis but also about the way that person would behave in the face of everyday life. It is only when people are truly imaginative and courageous that they seem to be compelling individuals. We see that those with imagination and courage are truly alive and are living their lives to the fullest. Then the question becomes, am I living an imaginative and courageous life? And if not, why not?

CURIOSITY

In some ways it seems a discussion about imagination and courage would come after curiosity, and yet, as an examination of the subject reveals, curiosity often depends on courage and imagination to proceed. Curiosity is a property of degree: we are all born curious, but in time our curiosity wanes. Curiosity is the spark that enables imagination to burn brightly.

We learn to think of curiosity as something that can be teased, nurtured and coaxed. Toddlers exhibit constant curiosity until they finally seem to surrender to requirements to *behave*. To be well-behaved, to exhibit self-control, for many people manifests in behavior that gives them the appearance of having no interests at all. Behaving is sitting still, remaining quiet. As toddlers master walking and the rudiments of language, they reach a point where their questions about anything and everything peak just as an impatient society searches for methods to turn their enthusiasm into manageable behavior. Some people have been so overly influenced by unintended efforts to diminish their curiosity that, for the rest of their lives, they act like the elephant who, on learning that his leg is chained to a stake, stops all attempts at trying to free himself, regardless of whether or not the chain is fastened to anything other than his leg. Fortunately, there are individuals whose curiosity runs so deep and strong that nothing seems to dampen it. These folks become the out-of-the-box thinkers who spend their lives trying to startle the rest of us awake. We find their names on the rolls of scientists, inventors, writers, artists, and thinkers within a whole range of enterprises where the property of curiosity is vital.

The property of time is an important feature of curiosity because it can serve as an instrument of social pressure, a tool for governing behavior. A "hurry-up" mentality can be destructive to one's sense of curiosity, and the effects can be long lasting. Moreover, place, change, regret, love, passion, fear, hatred, and memory each may affect the development and utility of curiosity. Time and place are critical components: If we are born into abject poverty, our curiosity will be dulled by hunger. If we live in a stultifying environment, a multitude of external factors may override our interests or prevent their development. Similarly, change or the lack of it may stimulate or thwart our attention. Our experiences with other people may enhance or hinder our curiosity in ways we understand emotionally, through love, passion, fear and hatred. But, regardless of our level of curiosity, our memory maintains a record of our experiences, and a re-examination of those experiences can rekindle the flame of our curiosity and awareness.

If we have the good fortune to be born into the right *place*, in a *time* of prosperity, to parents who are well educated, then our chances are good for growing up in a rich learning environment. Some have the added advantage of understanding Mihaly Csikszentmihalyi's notion that optimal learning experience involves "improving the content of experience" in a context of autonomy.[24] He writes, "The most important step in emancipating oneself from social controls is the ability to find rewards in the events of each moment. If a person learns to enjoy and find meaning in the ongoing stream of experience, in the process of living itself, the burden of social controls automatically falls from one's shoulders. Power returns to the person when rewards are no longer relegated to outside forces."[25]

Perhaps the greatest lesson of all is that the learning that enables our autonomy cannot be reduced to a simple formula, routinely applied.[26] Csikszentmihalyi goes on to tell us that knowing what to do is in and of itself not enough, that without consistency of action we are once again back where we started.[27] Thus, we may begin to regard curiosity as the one property of life that can have the most effect on all of the others. We can understand intuitively that a life without questions cannot provide answers, and that this condition leads to intellectual impoverishment. If we are to live lives that move us to maturity, we must not lose our inquisitiveness. We must remain in control of our mental faculties, and we must understand the dynamics of learning: that proportionate challenge is stimulating.[28]

Curiosity may be the one property that has enabled our species to survive in a world overwhelmed with change simply because it drives the process. The most important lesson about curiosity may be that strong interests are the primary stuff of autonomy and authenticity, which means that we do not create a real self until our interests move beyond ourselves. With this in mind, it may be useful to think of novelty as a rip or tear in the fabric of our cultural indoctrination. Thus, we may imagine novelty as a method and means for developing strong interests. When we find expression for those, we move to the next qualitative asset, creativity.

CREATIVITY

Like curiosity, the property of creativity is something we all have in some measure, and yet it's more easily activated than curiosity. Creativity can be learned and applied, whereas curiosity can be stimulated but not forced. When we think of creativity, we picture originality, divergent thinking, and the bringing into being of something that is new and in some way unique.

Taking a fresh approach to creativity, I choose to regard it as a way of distinguishing ourselves from others, even as we attempt to endear ourselves to them by means of our creations or by enabling them to see something that we deem is missing in their perspective. In this light, creativity has a relational or social aspect that is seldom appreciated as such until we comprehend the nature of creativity in the making of art.[29] By extending this appreciation for things that inspire us, we can behold simultaneously our individuality and connectedness; we can intuitively make the connection that reverence is a property we should come by naturally.

REVERENCE

Reverence is the point at which curiosity is brought up short, reduced to awe, some fashion of respect, or perhaps even fear. Reverence represents the outer bounds of our awareness, the edge of the abyss that separates the known from the unknowable. The term "reverence" appears most often in a religious context, but that's not my intention nor is it the primary usage Paul Woodruff has chosen for his book titled *Reverence: Renewing a Forgotten Virtue*. Woodruff writes, "Reverence begins in a deep understanding of human limitations; from this grows the capacity to be in awe of whatever we believe lies outside our control—God, truth, justice, nature, even death. The capacity for awe, as it grows, brings with it the capacity for respecting fellow human beings, flaws and all."[30]

Woodruff suggests it's a mistake to associate reverence solely with religion when it should instead be a property of community. He says we should not confuse reverence with respect, since reverence calls for respect only when it's due.[31] Woodruff's goal is to establish the concept of reverence as "the well-developed capacity to have the feelings of awe, respect, and shame when these are the right feelings to have."[32] He suggests that if we do not have the capacity for reverence then we are missing something of our humanity and that, absent that quality, "we cannot explain why we should treat the natural world with respect."[33]

Immanuel Kant, one of the most rigorous thinkers of the Enlightenment, reached the conclusion that there are spheres of life about which we are bound by our human limitations to remain hopelessly ignorant. To put it in terms familiar to us today, he determined that humans don't have the physical hardware to process the software of divinity or Divine knowledge. This was in part his justification for the concept of faith. In light of this recognition, and in the shadow of our ubiquitous human differences throughout the world, I can't think of a capacity of life more lacking or more appropriate for the twenty-first century than making the intellectual effort to truly appreciate and apply the property of reverence.

Reverence may indeed be a cornerstone of maturity. Moreover, a robust resurrection of the notion of reverence contains the essential ingredients for preventing clashes of faiths. Paul Woodruff puts it this way: "If you desire peace in the world, do not pray that everyone share your beliefs. Pray instead that they all be reverent."[34] For my own use of the term "reverence" I'm going to add the notion of the "sacred" and borrow the dictionary's definition as "worthy of respect." It doesn't matter whether you are devoutly religious, an agnostic or an atheist, the very least we owe one another as human beings on this planet is to treat everyone as if every single life is worthy of respect. In other words, reverence in both a religious and humanistic sense means that human lives are sacred. This is a conclusion I think most people can determine on their own if they take enough time to reflect about it. This brings us to solitude.

SOLITUDE

The September of life for many of us represents our first real opportunity to embrace large pools of solitude. Once characterized as a monkish virtue by the Scottish philosopher David Hume, solitude is certainly rare enough today to qualify as such. To experience solitude in the twenty-first century more often than not requires a deliberate attempt to override time, place, and our ever-changing mainstream media. It means turning off the telephone, computer, TV, radio, CD player, and our personal digital assistants and leaving them off until we can once again hear the echoes and reverberations of our own thoughts. Most of human thought occurs beneath consciousness, so it shouldn't be surprising that long periods of silence must produce intermittent floods of thoughtful contemplation. Insightful revelation can emerge if simply given a chance and the solitude to develop.

Throughout our lives we dream and search, reach and get. We become disillusioned or bored, and then we rethink and start the process over again. Later in life, most of the things that have occupied our lives as priorities begin to seem more and more like trivialities. We come to realize that what is truly important is that part of us which will linger after we are gone, whether it exists in the memories of others or through individual deeds that will outlive us. As Erik Erikson put it, "I am that which survives me."[35]

Unfortunately though, the tenor of our society is such that when we begin to act as if there is meaning to be sifted from experience, many of our peers will tend to resent it; they'll remind us at every opportunity of all of the quests for knowledge that have led to disaster. Those who refuse to try to better understand the world will spare no insult in their contempt for those who act as if learning really matters in enhancing quality of life. Moreover, there exists enough collective guilt and uncertainty about knowledge and wisdom to make all but the most confident of individuals feel that the effort to learn may indeed be an exercise in delusion.

An immersion in solitude and a reexamination of the properties of life mentioned here present a wonderful opportunity to study the hurried misunderstandings we've acquired. Through reflection we can better understand the human predicament and put our relations with others into perspective.

WISDOM

Wisdom is thought to be a pinnacle property of maturity. It is broadly defined to include insightfulness, enlightenment, sensibility, superior judgment, and the good sense to understand that sometimes wisdom sets itself apart from knowledge. Even though wisdom is often considered to be a part of common sense, it is also a characteristic of wisdom to see through common sense when the term stands for common illusion.

Throughout history, the wisest philosophers among us have pointed out that the property of wisdom comes with a built-in component of modesty and that when declarations of wisdom appear without reserve there may be reason to suspect otherwise. In addition, a desire for wisdom is more apt to produce it than knowledge gained simply because learning is expected.

I've always thought Socrates was a bit presumptuous and arrogant to declare that "the unexamined life is not worth living." He would have been on much firmer ground to have said something like, "The examined life increases in quality in direct proportion to the effort exerted." Taking the concept further, he might have said that a life without passion is unworthy, since the absence of passion probably would indicate little worthy of examination.

That Americans prize wisdom so little has always puzzled me. Perhaps because the founding fathers valued the pursuit of happiness so much as to state it boldly in the Declaration of Independence, we seem to miss the point about wisdom versus happiness. If we learn anything from philosophy, it is that the direct pursuit of happiness is a fool's journey and is virtually guaranteed to end in failure. Happiness derives from purpose, and purpose itself is a product of an effort engaged in for its own sake, not for the benefit of happiness. Purpose cannot be given to us; we must discover it for ourselves.

The property of wisdom appears throughout this book and may be considered a continuous means of addressing all of the other properties discussed. Moreover, it would seem to be the last on the list, were it not for the property of compassion, which I believe derives from wisdom.

COMPASSION

Most dictionary definitions of compassion portray it as a deep awareness of the suffering of others along with some kind of effort or intent to relieve it. In this way, compassion is, without a doubt, a property that can be developed through learning. Compassion, like reverence, is often thought to be a primary property of religion. Although I view it more broadly, my point is best made in that context. Roman Catholic priest Thomas Merton characterized compassion as "a keen awareness of the interdependence of all things."[36] Awareness is indeed an integral component of compassion.

Going even further, the tenets of Buddhism make

a compelling case that compassion is one property for which the world remains truly famished. It's becoming widely known, for instance, that only 20 percent of the world's population has enough material wealth to live above abject poverty and that the bottom 20 percent live in unimaginable squalor. Most people in the developed world guard themselves aesthetically from this travesty in part by remaining oblivious to it. At best, the affluent tend to deal with the issue superficially through a mild form of commiseration. This falls far short of the consideration necessary to address the problem with enough conviction to inspire real progress.

Simply put, compassion equals caring. People are dying for a lack of nourishment, not because of a scarcity of food, but, as the Buddhists suggest, because the world is starved of compassion. Empathy connects us to the plight of others, but empathy is only a feeling. When compassion is thought of as a property of life, it gains substance as a form of action.

In the West, we still harbor a popular fear (often beneath consciousness) of the concepts of altruism and altruistic behavior—a holdover from our ideological Cold War with the former Soviet Union. Anything that we do in a public context that appears overly generous raises suspicions about giving in to socialism. And yet, nearly a third of our economy is made up of nonprofit organizations comprising millions of people who work tirelessly to make the world a better place.

The XIV Dalai Lama and exiled spiritual leader of Tibet maintains that one of our primary human drives is the pursuit of happiness. Since this is the case, he says, compassion should be a dominant force in our lives and should therefore also be an attainable and teachable aspiration for humankind.[37]

He acknowledges that we also have the capacity for evil, but he believes that the latter tendency is subordinate to the former. In other words, even mean people pursue good most of the time.

For decades psychologists have been telling us that significant emotional events are also opportunities to make important changes in our lives. Changing something about our temperament or personality in an effort to become more compassionate, or even to change our course in life, can be an incredibly hard thing to do. Whenever I think about seemingly intractable problems, I'm reminded of Carl Sagan's introduction of wormholes into the genre of science-fiction novels.[38] Wormholes defy the common understanding of physics and offer access to other dimensions of time and place. They provide a rip in the fabric of time. The image of wormholes strikes a metaphorical chord with Viktor Frankl's experience as a prisoner in Auschwitz during World War II. He observed that, though few in number, there were always people in the concentration camps "comforting others, giving away their last piece of bread."[39] Frankl's observations of the best and worst examples of humanity enabled him to perceive of time in a way that resembles a perceptual wormhole, an empathetic connection in the fabric of humanity, an aperture through which urgency in a humanistic sense is so well defined that the things that really matter in life tower over the ones that don't. He says, "Live as if you were living already for the second time and as if you had acted the first time as wrongly as you are about to act now."[40] This is an intensely moving statement, and is close in analogy to a fissure in our ordinary discernment of time and place. The only way we are likely to make use of this breach in awareness, however, is through

flashes of insight and in moments of deep appreciation. Such instants resonate with the rapturous
experiences that accompany maturity.

The metaphysics of living with the level of atten-
tiveness Frankl asks of us may seem too hard
because of the fleeting way we perceive experience.
And yet, this is very much the approach I believe is
necessary when we contemplate slipping through,
wormhole fashion, into the aforementioned properties of life. These properties are open avenues of
experience, representing opportunities to distinguish the urgency of significance without the drama
and consequences of a powerfully emotional event,
but with very real prospects for improvement just
the same. You just have to approach them as if
insight is there for the taking and as if you are
determined enough to find an entrance that leads to
a new echelon of understanding.

A deep appreciation for all of life arises from a
wide-awake attunement to the life of the mind.
Indeed, how can we even use the phrase *life of the
mind* without acknowledging that without a mind
there is no life? We humans live in our heads, and
the quality of everything in our lives depends upon
what we do there. Everything we do in life, everything we see, everything we hear, and everything we
care about, hope for or aspire to, is mediated by the
quality of our thoughts and by our increasing ability to make compassionate choices and discriminat-
ing judgments. This level of awareness sheds new,
hopeful light on the human predicament.

Chapter Two

THE HUMAN PREDICAMENT

*Every excess causes a defect; every defect an
excess. Every sweet hath its sour;
every evil its good.*
—Ralph Waldo Emerson

L ife is full of contradictions. My friend and fellow author James R. Fisher, Jr., provides an
interesting example. He is an expert on organizational psychology but has never found an
organization where he fit in. Likewise Erik Erikson,
an orphan, wrote the book on identity, but his own
life experience suggests he didn't know who he was.
M. Scott Peck, author of the best-selling *The Road
Less Traveled,* actually took the familiar path of
wine, women, and song while he suggested that we
take another.[41] The most celebrated experts who
publish advice about relationships are often eligible
for the record books because of their number of
marriages. Those who preach love and friendship
are often cold and inaccessible to those who should
be closest to them. Those who teach compassion are
often cruel, and those who tell us how to calm and
still our lives are sometimes more uptight than we

are. Those who can see can't touch, I've often said, and those who can touch can't see. So it shouldn't come as a surprise for us to learn that people who have figured out how best to relate to others often feel absolved from the need to do so, since they think their contribution is made already by the observation. Moreover, people whose ability to relate is instinctive and on target to begin with are often hostile to theories about relating. As a result, this facet of life sometimes seems more mysterious than need be.

My search of the evidence in both psychology and neurology suggests that human beings are hardwired for contradiction because we have a split-brain architecture, or bicameral mind, as it's sometimes characterized. We are uniquely capable of adopting and holding on to irreconcilable ideas— ideas so incompatible that one should easily cancel the other, were it not for our capacity to isolate opposing beliefs within the corridors of our minds. In other words, we can hold contrary opinions in such a way that the inconsistency doesn't necessarily link up to reveal a discrepancy. Cognitive dissonance is a very real phenomenon, but we can often hold dissonance at bay, especially when the opposing ideas don't seem to be directly related.[42]

Our capacity for tolerating contradiction is so strong that it has the power to reshape memory. Mark Twain is said once to have quipped that the older he got, the more he remembered things that never happened. Friedrich Nietzsche put it this way: "'I have done that,' says my memory. 'I cannot have done that'—says my pride, and remains adamant. At last—memory yields."[43] My point is that self-deception undermines maturity, and the only way it can be overcome is to make a serious effort to see through it. As Janet Landman has observed, "The failed side of self-knowledge is self-deception."[44]

World literature is full of examples of characters who let their strengths also become their weaknesses because they lose perspective about how to balance their lives. To me, balance is an inadequate model for understanding how strengths become liabilities. A bit of the human contradiction resides in all of us, and the only way to turn it to our advantage is through gaining enough perspective to keep it from causing us to act in ways that defeat our better aspirations. Left unexamined, our contradictory nature has a tendency to ferment with despair and existential anxiety. Making wise choices is harder in practice than in theory, but, if one cannot recognize a wise choice even in theory, then one is doomed to a kind of ignorance that feeds upon itself.

I suspect our tendency to overlook the chasm between advice given and the nature of the giver is a holdover from the way most of us were schooled. We come to expect that someone who appears to have already figured out the solution to a problem will no longer be bothered by it, just as when you take a course in a particular subject and feel you are thereafter inoculated against having to do it again. Resolving the predicament of human contradiction is not that simple. Maturity involves developing the ability to see through our compulsion to deceive ourselves and being ever alert to the need to do so.

MORTALITY

As human beings, we are anxious by nature because we are mortal. In our accomplishments as individuals we may best Einstein's theory of relativity, cure cancer, or invent a communication medium more useful than the Internet. We may produce the kind of knowledge that literally saves the planet, but we are still going to die—each one of us—and soon. We already know from our examination of the property of time that human lifespans are pathetically short, although we willfully embrace illusions to the contrary. Even the calendar we use to measure time helps to hide the reality of our finite lives. We are comforted by the seemingly endless Mondays, Fridays, and Sundays available to us and insulated from the truth that each one of these days is unique, never to be repeated, and could be our last. Death awaits each and every one of us, but our mental apparatus gives us the capacity to ignore the fact as a means of quieting our anxiety about it.

The danger of overindulging in this form of self-deception is that the anxiety comes back disguised as something annoying but less threatening. We delude ourselves that situations and other people are obstacles to our happiness, when in reality these distractions simply serve to mask our greatest fears. It's the certainty of death that stands in our way. Somewhere beneath our consciousness lies the haunting scrap of dissonance that, except for having only a finite amount of time on earth, each of us might live long enough to achieve wealth, fame, nirvana, or whatever goal we might deem worthy of the effort.

Some people scoff at the suggestion that existential angst even exists. Some cultures have other names for this kind of anxiety, but none are free from its effects. Moreover, it doesn't matter whether you are religious, agnostic, or atheist, mortality causes apprehension, whether we choose to acknowledge it or not. Our anxiety intensifies with the realization that, regardless of our affection for fairness, society's deck is stacked: advantage falls to the few born during the *right time,* in the *right place,* and to the *right parents,* which no close reading of the state of the world can deny.

Being aware of the fact that our actions often reflect the contradictory nature of our minds doesn't automatically help us resolve our dilemmas. That we are physically and mentally rigged for self-deception seems to contribute to our fascination with tragedy. A disaster that does not personally involve us can be evidence that our luck still holds. Many of us also take comfort in the idea of transcending our physical bodies in death, if only through metaphor, which brings us to the metaphysics of soul.

Author Tom Wolfe once suggested in an interview that the best definition of soul is the sum of one's human relations. This struck me as a very profound statement and one that needs to be greatly expanded. It's useful to think of soul not just as the metaphoric sum of one's human relations but also as a model applicable to all relations. In other words, we can think of soul as the sum of our relating to people and to everything and anything one can relate to. This way, a person's life can be thought of as a project, as a piece of art, a work in progress, a spark in a dark void, something worth doing. If you give it your all, here and now, you have nothing to fear at the end.

People of diverse cultures have myriad ways of perceiving and expressing ideas about the existence and nature of the human soul. But, if we begin with the notion that spirituality emerges from this soulful relating, then we have something concrete to talk about, regardless of our position on the reality of souls or on the question of whether there is life after death.

RELATIONSHIPS AND RELATING

Existentialist philosopher Søren Kierkegaard argued that our unconscious despair is something that we can't rid ourselves of. You can't analyze or meditate it away, and you can't remove it with therapy. Anxiety and despair are part of the human condition.[45] This is what makes our beliefs about soul and spirituality so compelling and why understanding such despair is so important.

Our attempts to avoid despair and to soothe our individual selves through shared beliefs are aggravated, even threatened, by those people who do not agree with our take on reality. In other words, our doubts have a way of evolving into contempt for those who see the world differently than we do. It's as if the ferment of our anxiety and despair seethes beneath our consciousness, redirecting itself into disdain for anyone who would cast doubt on our hopes and thus confirm our greatest fears. What could threaten our sense of well-being more than exposure of our worldview as a facile, self-serving illusion?

To think that one person or group is spiritual and another is not is to miss the point entirely. To imagine that your soul is saved and another's is lost is blasphemy in both a religious and secular context, precisely because it is an act of misrelating. As we've seen, human beings are hardwired for contradiction, which makes our beliefs about ourselves worth careful scrutiny. Our deepest anxiety as human beings exists mostly at a subconscious level: it's a wretchedness Kierkegaard described as "despair unaware that it is despair," and as such it is the fuel that drives contempt.[46] This state cannot be overcome through a twelve-step program. As philosopher Rick Roderick once put it, "You can't be cured of what it is that you are."[47]

Thus, we must be very careful and aware of our inborn tendency to camouflage our fears and existential doubts about the world with a focus on the apparent social and lifestyle deviations of others. What starts with pointing out little differences often ends with one person or group thinking there is no room for the other. This is the antithesis of relating and is totally void of soul and spirituality. One need only remember Adolph Hitler's Nazi regime, or Bosnia and Rwanda, or Osama bin Laden. Obtaining anything near objectivity in understanding our nature is impossible without an examination of the properties of life as they relate to all cultures and not just our own.

A comprehension of human relations cannot be complete, however, unless it includes an understanding of how we relate to material possessions. Just as objects in space warp time, so do our possessions twist our relationships with others. We tend to cluster in social circles with those of similar material wealth and rarely, if ever, come in contact with those who are very far above or below our level of prosperity. Moreover, throughout the trajectory of our lives, our relationship with material possessions will change within the context of time and place. The importance we attach to material wealth will wax and wane at intervals until—should we be fortunate enough to live so long—we reach a point where the very term "property" is meaningless. Most of us acquire deep psychological attachments to artifacts and keepsakes passed down to us through parents and grandparents. If we lose these items, or if something happens to them, we may experience despair and grief as intense as if someone had died. What's really at issue here is not the loss of these things per se but the underlying impermanence their loss implies. For indeed, given time, all of these articles will someday wind up in a landfill or a scrap heap of one kind or another.

Maturity demands that we sort through the psychological aspects of real property because, until we do, all of our human relationships will remain distorted by the gravity of acquisitiveness. In America in particular, our great wealth can be an obstacle to objectivity. In *The Soul of Capitalism,* William Greider puts our dilemma in perspective, saying, "The point of overwhelming abundance is now plainly in our face and beyond argument, yet seldom discussed as the new central premise of the economic condition. The incompleteness at the core of American life, I believe, is also about this new fact of history. Our situation is unique—learning how to live amid endless plenty and, ironically, how to live well in spite of it. Our ancestors never had to face such a struggle. We cannot escape it."[48]

As social animals we are so warped by materiality that, although no one likes to admit it, our success is sometimes enhanced when our friends fail, and our pleasure diminished when they succeed. Philip Slater said it best: "Once people get the idea that there isn't enough of something, they begin to deprive each other of what there is."[49]

Eighty percent of the world's populations are poor, and the bottom 20 percent are so poor that their plight is nearly unmentionable among the 20 percent who have ready access to material necessities. Only under enormous pressure will the mainstream media make a serious effort to explain the ethical contradictions of abject poverty in the shadow of grand affluence and among people who view themselves as architects of moral virtue.

Economic materiality is so forcefully promoted by our culture that our economic success as a society depends upon the certainty that we will cheerfully purchase things we don't need, even if they are proven dangerous to our health and to the environment in which we live. The gap between rich and poor, though deplorable, may not be as disturbing as the fact that most of the people who are considered financially successful are mired in the gravity of acquisitiveness, unable to see that, beyond a baseline of physical and material comfort, the quest for more wealth is itself a recipe for unhappiness. Indeed, where material gain is concerned, ambition and happiness are tenuously compatible aspirations: having one tends to inhibit the other. Millions of people strive to accumulate possessions unaware that it is not the goods themselves they seek, but status. The goods stand in where richness of relationship is lacking.

Reconciling the world's enormous material wealth and its arbitrary geographic distribution is a dissonant endeavor. There are times when it takes great care not to develop contempt for the very things that make our lives comfortable. This paradox came to me decades ago during the Cold War. I was attending Stanford University's professional publishing course and was sharing a dormitory with journalists from the then-Soviet Union. One of my proudest moments as a citizen of the United States was when we took these guests to a supermarket. One of the Russians got so excited over the seemingly endless supply of bananas that he talked about it for days. It's still a fond memory, but since then I've been keenly aware that there are many people from the poorest nations in the world with whom I would be embarrassed to visit a typical

American grocery store. Not because we have so much, but because they have so little.

Mind you, I don't want to suggest that I don't like nice things, fine clothes, useful appliances, cutting-edge technology, good food, fine restaurants, and all of the material comforts that enrich our lives. Just broaching this subject is often enough to incur accusations of being a bleeding heart. In the face of such derision, my response is simply this: Regardless of who you are or where you live in the world, if you don't deal with the problem of global poverty and human starvation with some level of intellectual honesty, then you cannot lay claim to moral high ground in any sense of the term. Moreover, if you see yourself as being an otherwise very spiritual person, then you are fooling yourself. Someday your self-deception is going to show itself in a form of anxiety that is completely misplaced and just as likely misattributed.

Clearly, values define a culture. A misalignment of values can lead to misrelating among nations, among groups, and among individuals within a group. At the same time, relating is a core concern of humankind.

In a passage that the late Rick Roderick described as one of the densest in all of philosophy, Kierkegaard fashioned an esoteric argument that spirit is self, but a self is not a relation. Rather, self is a synthesis, and despair is but a misrelating of synthesis, a sickness of the spirit.[50] A self is a self only because there is an entity known as the other. An inward journey is meaningless without a fundamental appreciation of the outer world of knowledge. There is no point in making the trip, if nothing will be found when we get there.

Using the term "spirituality" to represent the

qualitative sum of human relating offers much more than today's popular attempts to embrace the mystical peculiarities of an imagined spirit world. Spirituality as a measure of human relationships offers us a principled compass for the creation of a better world here. For idealists and materialists alike, a world in which relationships embody aspirations for universal improvements in relating would truly be a spiritual place to live.

Looked at in this way, supernatural metaphysics aside, soul becomes a measure of existence that can unquestionably survive one's death. The works, deeds, and human relations we leave behind can and will exist in the memories of those who survive us as a contribution to their successes in life. Great deeds and great relationships foster great souls.

MISRELATING

It has become a cliché, or perhaps a runaway meme, to say that differences among people should be celebrated. I've said so myself on more than one occasion. It just strikes a virtuous chord in the minds of tolerant people to imagine celebrating distinctions. But a better approach, and indeed a more pragmatic and mature approach, is to concentrate on minimizing the differences among us.

The reality of human relationships on a global scale is that, no matter what we believe or how altruistic or how unselfish we are, we can be sure that there are people somewhere on the planet who disagree with our worldview. They disagree with such vehemence that they would consider killing us rather than tolerate our views.

In *Beyond the American Dream*, I tried to surgically slice through the dilemma that divides the development of conscience and the willingness to stand up for one's beliefs from the tolerance necessary to sustain a democracy. A good life calls for commitment and tolerance, but in troubled societies this reality slams up against the certainty that tolerance, in most of us, can be stretched to the breaking point. History is clear about this. There are things worth dying for, but at times it seems beyond the pale of philosophers to articulate just what these things are.

Democracy itself is supposed to be a relief valve for disagreement, but it doesn't always work: the American Civil War is a case in point. Absent such examples as lessons, we tend to view the peoples of the world as having reaped what they deserve. And yet, this "just world hypothesis" is the mere tip of the iceberg. Not only do we look upon the world with a predetermined and wholly internalized sense of justice that automatically adjusts our expectations based on our judgments about other people, but also we seesaw between sympathy and tacit pleasure at the misfortunes of others. We've only to look beneath the superficiality of our worldview and examine the basis for our judgments of others to have our heretofore unacknowledged philosophy of relating to others thrown into stark relief. The Germans have a word for pleasure in the suffering of others: *Schadenfreude*. Scholars differ widely on the presupposition of malice that derives from *Schadenfreude*. Some see it as mere comeuppance; others see it as sadistic pleasure, but the fact that we do not have a word for it in English does not mean that it does not exist in our culture.

From childhood we are measured with a set of expectations as to how to behave in the world, and this cultural conditioning lasts a lifetime. We learn to regard those who do not measure up as being subject to correction. So, when others commit crimes, we expect them to be punished. When they spend foolishly, we expect that they *ought* to be broke. But when they take financial risks and win, our response may still be contempt, however elaborately disguised. The more competitive the society, the greater its psychic investment in the success or failure of others.

When the World Trade Center towers were destroyed in September of 2001, Americans were outraged. Justice, to most of us, meant annihilation of those responsible for killing thousands of innocent people. We were in no mood to consider alternative views. This feeling was so strong that the public was willing to overlook the fact that our bombs dropping on Afghanistan to defeat the Taliban were also killing innocent people. The ease with which we discount the value of others when our own lives are threatened is the fuel of genocide.

No attempt at education is ever enough that does not focus on human relations on a global scale. We can't really learn what kind of people we are until we ask ourselves a multitude of questions concerning the fortune of others. Do the people on this planet who are at this moment starving to death deserve such a fate? What would the founders of the world's great religions say to us when we stand aside and turn our heads from those who are dying in the shadow of our enormous wealth and military power? Do people who have no health insurance deserve to go untreated? Are the people around the world who work for pennies a day—to provide goods that we want but don't really need—treated fairly? Are people who earn a minimum wage justly compensated? Does everyone reap what he or she sows? Do people who take a life deserve to have theirs forfeited? Will the edict of "an eye for an eye" make the whole world blind, as Mahatma Gandhi said it would?

American culture has become so absorbed in the throes of our economic system that millions of us have internalized a worldview laden with market values as the measure to value all valuations. Every problem is viewed as having an economic cause and solution. We believe the incessant propaganda that individuals and businesses of all stripes will not act—*ever*—without monetary incentive, specifically tax incentives, for any reason. We ignore the fact that the work of volunteers accounts for a significant share of our economy.

One of the most important lessons to be gleaned from history about relating is that any and all arguments targeted at the visceral level of our relationships can and will incur an unreasoned response on the part of those who have been attacked and that this part of our nature is what political propagandists depend on to achieve their agendas, especially during elections. In other words, they rely upon our propensity for misrelating, fully understanding that it takes an extraordinary effort for most people to rise above it. Misrelating is driven by a human frailty that often manifests itself thus: The fewer the facts, the stronger the opinion; the stronger the opinion, the greater the emotion. The greater the emotion, the sooner will volatility reach a point where any measure is acceptable for stamping out the "other."

Individuals who are deemed incapable of relating are characterized by us as psychopaths, and the darkest measure of misrelating by whole societies, one against the other, is evidenced in times of war, when we dehumanize and demonize others to a point where they are said to be unworthy of living.

The history of infamous acts of evil in the world offers clear examples of misrelating—of ignorance taken to an extreme stage of malignancy—antihuman and thus anti-intellectual to the core of our species. What I aim to make clear is that the only force powerful enough to deal with the inhuman effects of misrelating is the conscious and self-aware application of goodwill.

Without an extraordinary effort to reason our way through the effects of our relationships with others, we exhibit immature behavior by following our instincts to look after ourselves and our own. Our biological predisposition for favoring small groups is necessary for our social well-being, and yet for the good of humanity it needs to be amended.[51] We favor family by putting our own children first. While it seems intuitively wise to seek advantage for them, there are many cases where these acts not only are self-defeating, but also are degrading to our children, ourselves and the others over whom we've sought advantage. Examples of this kind of behavior are ubiquitous, but I need give only one to make the point—that of the parent who uses his company's high-tech shop to create his child's science project.[52]

Misrelating is humankind's most pressing problem. It always has been, and perhaps it always will be so. The quality of life in each and every generation depends upon our efforts to better understand one another. Moreover, misrelating is a problem for which a graduate education to become a "professional" hasn't much to offer in the way of remedy. In his book *Disciplined Minds*, Jeff Schmidt has shown that the psychological effects of graduate school often render "professionals" even more susceptible than high school graduates to supporting militant actions toward others.[53]

It's sad but unalterably true that, in time, all human relationships unravel and disintegrate—whether through life changes or simply because of the aging process itself. Seniors who've written about the experience of this unraveling tell us that a large part of the ability to cope with this reality comes from not being surprised by it. Far more important is to possess a determination to get beyond it, a topic to be explored in Chapter Four.

AGING AND DESPAIR

Human longevity has increased dramatically in the last century. And yet, from Alaska to Florida, and from Baja to Maine, senior citizens by the hundreds of thousands are being warehoused in nursing homes and shot full of anesthetizing chemicals to keep them still and quiet. This is an ugly matter that doesn't get nearly the attention it should.

In my twenties and thirties I was reluctant to discuss the inevitability of death, even in a hypothetical sense. But somewhere near or during my early fifties, I began to notice more and more people who not only were willing to discuss death but also were somewhat comforted by the shadow it casts, myself included. I'm not morbid about it nor do I dwell on it excessively, but shadow is precisely the right metaphor to describe the sensation. It's like knowing that death is close by, and its presence is a gentle but pressing reminder that one should make the extra effort to sort out what is really important and let the lesser things go. A simple but practical voice inside one's head begins to whisper subtle reminders like, "This super-warranted hammer you've just purchased at Sears is very likely the last one you will ever need to buy." Or, when considering a new car, "I wonder if it will last longer than my ability to drive?"

Sometimes I think it strange that the fear of death has remained so ubiquitous throughout time and regardless of place. To die is simply to go back to the state of wasn't, back to the time of before we were, so to speak. Because we are here now, we have no sense of then, although we were dead during all of the time before we came into being. Upon much reflection I've come to believe that humans' greatest fear about death is not the terror of nothingness, but the dread of remorse about all of the things we won't know, the events we will not witness, and the joys we will miss. The knowledge about all of the great triumphs, trials, and tribulations ahead for humankind, and the great questions: Will other life be found in the universe? How will life on earth end? Will a giant asteroid hit our planet? Will all diseases be cured? Will machines do all of the work in the future? Will our great-great-grandchildren live for 200 years? Will human beings ever learn to get along without war? Will the world ever be truly civilized?

Not knowing is the horror of nonexistence. And yet, how do we square this insight with the reality that so many of us strive to learn so little and squander so many opportunities during our brief lives? The notion of impermanence has profound psychological effects in both our conscious and unconscious lives. If we were to learn that the earth will be destroyed by a gigantic asteroid in 200 years, we would likely be haunted by the prospect, even though it would occur long after we are gone.

Every few years the aspirations of a whole generation die out, dissipating like embers in a fireplace, forever reduced to ashes. This phenomenon of lost potential reminds me of some of my all-time favorite movie lines and scenes. In *Blade Runner*, for instance, Rutger Hauer plays a human replicant who has tasted life. Lamenting his experiences in memory and the inevitability of his own death, he says, "All those moments will be lost in time like tears in rain." Near the end of *Dr. Zhivago*, the general who speculates on what has happened to Lara refers to her as "a nameless number on a list that was afterwards mislaid." And finally, in a voiceover by Robert Redford at the close of *A River Runs Through It*, the narrator speaks of being alone in the half-light of the canyon. Speculating about the essence of the natural world, he says he is "haunted by waters." These statements carry a sense of overwhelming finality that causes them to sort of hang in the air after they are spoken aloud. They have a dark side for sure, but they also call attention to the profundity of existence and the possibilities presented in the here and now. Each generation that's born and dies has its share of successes and failures and much that is worthy of being passed on. The finality of death is for so many of us too late a realization of prospects lost. As long as we are alive, we still have an opportunity to live a life that really matters.

A tragic history of misrelating and the dark side of aging aside, the evidence of our continued propensity to thrive as a species is straightforward confirmation that the good human beings do outnumber the bad. But for mainstream media's fascination with the negative side of life, this would never be in doubt. Every day there are billions of acts of kindness and self-sacrifice perpetrated by millions of people whose desire to do something good in the world provides its own intrinsic reward. People *en masse* donate their money, their time, and even their bodily organs to strangers for the sheer joy of doing something worthwhile. If the motivation for good did not surpass the will for evil, our species would have perished long ago.

MOTIVATION

In their book *Human Givens*, Joe Griffin and Ivan Tyrrell say this about motivation: "Without motivation human beings cannot find meaning in what they do and are left wandering feebly in the joyless grey limbo between a healthy, fulfilling life and insanity."[54] I can relate to this.

During the start-up days of the Prudhoe Bay oil field, I had a job as technician on Alaska's North Slope. It was exciting work, and the pay was extraordinarily high. The oil field was 800 miles from where I lived, so each week I flew to work via a company jet and then back home for a week off. My formal education to this point amounted to a high school GED and a few classes in police science and administration. I felt incredibly lucky at the time to have such a job and eventually was promoted into a management position despite my lack of a college degree.

The downside of this arrangement was that the work environment came with an authoritative organizational style, led in many cases by supervisors with extensive military experience. Our quarters at Prudhoe Bay were private rooms in a barracks-like hotel, and we ate our meals in the cafeteria. This meant workers shared meals with the managers. Having already served in the Marines and with a paramilitary police department, I gradually became more and more resentful of what I concluded were exhibitions of arbitrary power by individuals who, in my opinion, didn't deserve to be in management.

In time it developed that, for no conscious reason and without any deliberate plan, I began to read lots of newspapers and news magazines during my weeks off. Then, not realizing my unconscious agenda, I began asking, at the dinner table, questions of particular supervisors about current events. These were questions I was already sure they were unlikely to be able to answer. In effect, I became a self-appointed Socrates, determined to expose the fools in charge. I was very subtle, and to the best of my knowledge they never caught on, but then, I didn't realize what I was up to myself until much later. In hindsight, though, I can plainly see that it wasn't only retaliation that I was looking for by publicly revealing the ignorance of those whose authority I resented. My little game was a product of boredom and a desire not to be limited at mealtime to conversation about work—twelve hours a day was enough talk about that.

The end result of this experience was profound in effect and life-changing in scope: My interest in current events expanded into the study of myriad subjects and immersion in philosophy. It took me from the early George Wallace to Mahatma Gandhi. My smoldering curiosity burst into an all-out passion for lifelong learning that has not let up to this day. Granted, this is not a story of inspiration to be especially proud of, but it's true, and it contains a message critical for understanding the motivation for learning. The lesson is this: The reasons for learning and the methods involved are for many people not nearly as important as reaching a critical mass of knowledge where the satisfaction gained, in and of itself, is not only its own reward but also sufficient to keep the momentum going.

In the early years of my drive for self-education, I became obsessed with the mechanics of motivation for learning. I spent months reading and comparing divergent views about what prompts some people to learn continuously while others instead seem to be preoccupied with a need for constant entertainment devoid of meaningful content. No definite explanation emerged. Even today the battle continues among educational theorists for developing a model that nails learning theory to the wall. I gave up comparing theoretical models when I realized a simple truth: We make the effort to learn *whatever we really care about.*

When you care deeply about something, the motivation to learn about it will follow, free of any other psychological charges. Those of us with many years of experience don't need someone to tell us that we are motivated to learn what we already care about, but this is an incredibly insightful bit of knowledge we can pass on to younger generations. By what measure of logic should it be considered normal that young people pursue a subject or career field they don't really care about, only to become confused and bewildered when they don't have enough enthusiasm to continue their studies or take pleasure in their work? Why do we let this happen?

Many of the champions of alternative education were themselves recipients of a traditional education that they resented. Still, they managed to get far enough along to ignite their intellect in some fashion. The dynamics of reaching a critical mass of learning are easy to understand. One has only to consider the difficulty in learning how to read. In the beginning, the process can be both tedious and grueling. Once mastered, however, reading is its own reward. It's the same with hobbies. When people amass enough knowledge about a subject that interests them, they quickly reach a point where the pleasure of discovery is self-reinforcing. Then, once their intense interests are recognized by others, they receive even further reinforcement that reaches to the very core of their identity.

A passion for learning leads to a passion for life. Young people should be encouraged to develop deep interests, and adults should help them connect those interests to a broader exploration of the world. The very notion of maturity implies completion, and most of the things we finish with enthusiasm are born of significance. We cannot lead interesting lives without being interested in life, and, without strong interests, there is no path that leads to maturity.

LANGUAGE AND VALUES

As we learn to speak, we are introduced to language and a system of metaphors that enable us to understand one thing from having understood another. In this way we develop an arsenal of ideas that serve as props within our consciousness, presenting a background on which we are able to build and expand for the rest of our lives. We begin this process early in life by stitching ideas together through spatial mapping. In doing so, we come to understand that happiness means up and sadness means down. We learn that time is something we have, that it can be taken from us, that it has a trajectory, that it flows, and that it is equivalent to money. We learn that there are negative similarities among low, poor, bad, and down, and that the whole concept of morality relies upon accounting metaphors in which there are debts, payments, balances, and repayments.[55]

In response, we internalize a metaphorical credit-debit system to keep track of life's properties. We learn that important is big, that affection is warmth, that intimacy is closeness, that both life and love can be thought of as journeys, that "seeing is touching," that emotional effect is physical contact, that life has the attributes of a container, that our eyes are containers for our emotions, that vitality is substance, that life itself is "a game of chance," and that "seeing is understanding."[56] We learn that the same words and metaphors that apply to war (recall the word *arsenal* at the beginning of this discussion) will also serve to set the very tone and tenor that gives an argument context. This clearly suggests that people who are unaware of such intricacies can be easily manipulated.[57]

The language acquisition process that shapes a large part of what we believe about the world is nearly invisible, and yet it is readily apparent to anyone who will simply give it a hard look. Nevertheless, most people live out their whole lives without giving the dynamics of these forces a second thought. We take the sense of reality dictated by this cultural orientation as real and right to such a degree that we have no doubts that our own culture has reality pegged and every other differing culture simply has it wrong. What should really arrest our attention is that this is something all cultures do—each assumes superiority over others—which should jolt us into recognizing the subjectivity of our own views. We don't have reason to question the fact that an argument might be comparable to war, but what if in someone else's metaphors an argument represented a dance or a party?[58] The perspective would likely be a startling contrast to ours and one that suggests we may have the short end of the stick (another metaphor suggesting small is not as good as big).

My point here is not to engage in a protracted academic exposition about language but simply to make clear that a quest for knowledge requires a thorough examination of things most people assume were settled in grade school but which are, in an epistemological sense, as arbitrary as they are subjective. This kind of inquiry is critical to both maturity and authenticity. We should never lose sight of the fact that the properties of life brought to bear in this discussion rest upon a metaphorical foundation. That foundation must be examined brick by brick if we are to rise above the indifference routinely accepted as normal by all cultures who do not themselves engage in this process.

As our great literature demonstrates, human beings are champions of self-deception, especially in matters where our well-being conflicts with the interests and well-being of others. The average person is a genius when it comes to the creation of self-enhancing illusions. Perhaps the most fortunate thing about the human condition is that learning our way through pretentiousness takes us to higher levels of reasoning. When our knowledge reaches critical mass, it becomes a reward in its own right and is thus one of the most pleasurable things we can experience. On the other hand, the greatest tragedy may be that many people never realize the pleasure to be had from significant learning for the simple reason that they never make a serious effort to understand things for themselves. It's much more comfortable to believe that matters of the *heart* have nothing to do with the *head*—a metaphor that implies feeling is always a greater good than thinking.

Individuals who choose reason over the dictates of emotion are often ridiculed or dismissed for wanting to discuss unsettled questions or for acting too cerebral. Yes, reason has limits, which are evident in the perpetual debate among academics over what is and isn't knowable. Those matters aside, members of the general population typically prefer to avoid any of the hard questions of life, and many will go to great lengths to change the topic. If the issue is unanswerable, such as the true nature of the Divine, then changing the subject might be practical. But when the concern is over domestic, political, or philosophical questions about how we are to live, then dismissing the subject is irresponsible.

Such anti-intellectualism occurs, in part, because the very nature of learning is generally misunderstood. Much of the learning we achieve as human beings occurs beneath consciousness. To function in the world, for example, the fundamental learning we need is often acquired through osmosis. Lion cubs who've followed their mother on occasional hunts need no formal tests to see if they have been paying attention. They take in the learning they need after a few simple demonstrations. Similarly, we learn how to speak, how to get along with others (or not), how to judge character, and so forth through observation and total involvement. We become so astute at matching and picking up on patterns that throughout our lives we will make connections among disparate situations without having the slightest idea how we come by such understanding.[59]

Here is where confusion really starts to set in. A strange look on a playmate's face in a sandbox at age three, accompanied by a certain type of behavior that's reinforced again and again throughout childhood but never remembered, becomes a learned experience that later yields strong feelings about others. As adults we may interpret these feelings as being "intuitive." But, as John Stuart Mill is said to have argued, just because we don't remember learning something doesn't mean it's intuitive. An insight that appears to bypass reason may still have its roots in brain function. In point of fact, how could it be otherwise? Some of the most important actions we take in life are instinctive, lightning fast, and appear devoid of thought, but had we not at an earlier time internalized these options as possible courses of action, they would be unavailable to us in emergencies. Much of the critical learning we do in life stems from osmosis, but the gray matter in our heads is always involved.

As mentioned earlier, one of our most cherished metaphors is viscerally anti-intellectual, so much so that we relegate everything that truly matters to us to the heart. But, contrary to Aristotle's great wisdom (he attributed capabilities of the brain to the heart), the human heart does nothing more than function as a pump for the flow of blood. Regardless of what we say, or with how much passion we say it, matters of the heart occur in the *head*. Emotion is our source of passion; it makes life worthwhile. To relegate it to an organ that can't think makes no sense, unless we are trying to escape accountability for our actions.

Knowledge of consequence occurs to us through the perpetual pursuit of insight. Why, then, do so many people devalue, or even hate, those who search for meaningful knowledge beyond what is accepted as common sense? Our history shows that the error of popular sentiment is far more prevalent than the ubiquity of profound truths. If it is not because of fear or hatred, why do those of us who linger in the shadows in search of greater understanding incur so much derision from those who satiate their curiosity with willful illusions? If the search for knowledge is truly a journey (another common metaphor), and if we really expect to learn from experience, why do we hold our leaders in contempt when we find that they have changed a position over time? Do we think they should have been born with the truth and can't be trusted if their learning ever causes them to change their minds?

Once we begin to appreciate how we adopt the metaphors that express our take on reality, we also begin to better appreciate those whose experience leads them to view the world differently than we do. The implication is this: If we want to change our lives, we must change our metaphors. For example, if we truly think time is more precious than wealth, then we must stop speaking the language that time is money. If we really want to pursue truth for the sake of authenticity, then we must acknowledge that matters of the heart occur in the head, and we must act and think accordingly. To do otherwise is to act as if we are powerless where matters of the heart are concerned. The heart as the emotional center for humans is a lovely expression; it's poetic, romantic, and comforting. But, when the goal is to make the world a better place, this image is a major distraction and an impediment to progress in relating. If we really want to better understand ourselves, we must explore the very nature of understanding and how we comprehend one concept through the aid of others. Simply put, we must become our own language archaeologists and frequently pilfer the boneyard of language and dead metaphors.

For thousands of years, religious leaders have warned their followers of the perils that come with seeking forbidden knowledge, which they claim man is incapable of understanding. For more than two centuries, historians have spoken of the Enlightenment

as a period where the open-ended search for knowledge gave rise to modernity. In more recent years,
French intellectuals engaged in a school of thought
frequently referred to as postmodernism have made
some progress in demonstrating the futility of
absolute interpretation of texts.⁶⁰ The results of this
contentious dialog have prompted some people to fall
back to the earlier position that, in fact, man is incapable of ultimate knowledge and thus exploration
should not be pushed too far. In *The Twilight of
American Culture,* Morris Berman put this dilemma
into perspective: "The postmodern rebellion against
fixed forms finally leaves a positive legacy: Beware of
fixed forms. Yes, it was a sledgehammer to crack a
nut, but let us give credit where credit is due."⁶¹

Bursting the bubble of textual absolutes in no
way diminishes the search for knowledge—meaningful knowledge in particular. The lesson to be learned
from postmodernism, in my view, is simply to leave
the door of interpretation ajar (which history proves
beyond doubt is a wise thing to do); it makes a compelling case for cracking the code of our own cultural pretentiousness. To make progress as a society,
we surely must break through the barrier that causes millions of people to boast about their lack of
knowledge and to take pride in remaining ignorant.
In other words, we must make the case that anti-
intellectualism is an absurd strategy for living a fulfilling life.

It's a strange paradox when you give it some
thought. We tend to view primitive or Stone Age cultures as lacking intelligence. But, as Jared Diamond
points out in his book *Guns, Germs, and Steel*, the
reverse is likely to be true.⁶² A primitive environment
demands much more of individuals than does an
industrialized society, even though this seems

somewhat counterintuitive. I don't think it's an exaggeration to imagine that primitive human beings could derive as much edification from the landscape as we get from reading a chapter in a book.

In contemporary America large groups of people can, in effect, withdraw from society without becoming conspicuous. They may avoid voting or participating in civic or social functions. In primitive societies, on the other hand, all members who reached maturity were expected to use their intelligence in order to contribute to the good of the whole.[63] Imagine the improbability of finding members of a hunter-gatherer society who expressed pride in their lack of knowledge about hunting and food preparation. Contemporary American anti-intellectualism is no less ridiculous; we've just learned to accept it as normal. It's the standard way of life among people who value certitude more than exploration.

PEER POWER

In the 1950s, David Riesman characterized a large part of the American population as being "other-directed."[64] In the simplest sense, being other-directed means that a person looks to others for direction. People who are other-directed are heavily influenced by external authority, which includes *peer pressure*. When we hear the term "peer pressure," most of us think of the adolescent kind. How convenient: as adults we pretend to be no longer influenced by the opinions of others, yet the very notion of culture is laden with templates for oppressive scrutiny from one's peers.

On one hand, the opinions of others can diminish our individuality; on the other, they can lead to the kind of behavior that makes us think we live in a great country. We grow up internalizing the expectations of others with such force and intensity that, in time, we come to believe these convictions are our own and that we have arrived at them through deliberate, critical, and judicious analysis. So, it's not surprising at this stage in our development that we are no longer aware of the external pressures that prescribe how we are to live, eat, sleep, dress, work, and act. We've internalized them. But, if we cross too far over the line in our individual behavior, we are sure to experience the pressure anew. We have only to mistakenly wave at a stranger to feel a sudden flush of embarrassment.

Of course, peer pressure has a strong positive component. It provides the social cohesion that allows the very development of communal affiliation. But peer power as an extrinsic force is a lot like radiation: a little goes a long way. There are people our peers don't think we should associate with, stores in which neither rich nor poor people want to be seen shopping, books and magazines we would rather not be caught reading, and a vast array of clothing and jewelry one wouldn't want to be caught dead or even buried in. This is not to say that we should be oblivious to social concerns or that we should never care about what others think. Scratch beneath the surface of expected behavior, however, and peer pressure will reveal itself with a vengeance. This brings us to peer poverty.

Peer poverty occurs when people lose their sense of self, or worse, never develop intrinsic motivation or reasons for acting of their own volition, in favor of following the continuous, unrelenting demands of others. The consequences of peer poverty were among playwright George Bernard Shaw's greatest fears, namely to live an inauthentic existence and discover near the end of your life that you'd lived solely for the inane and selfish reasons of others.[65] The pain of this disclosure, he feared, would bedevil you till the end of your days, haunting you with the notion that you could have gone anywhere, been anything, and done anything but for a simple understanding of the dynamics of peer pressure.

The cosmic clock is ticking, but it's never too late to learn the lesson reflected in Ralph Ellison's *Invisible Man,* that paying the price of attention, with a sustained effort at understanding and comprehending the world and our place in it, is a requisite for a living a meaningful life. If we achieve such independence of thought, we ensure the respect of our peers long after we are gone. And this is peer power at its best. The heroes of our history stand out most often, not because they conformed to the peer pressures of their day, but because they rose to the occasion and set new and higher standards. Their actions and deeds reveal the value, importance, and responsibility for thinking beyond the impulse of peer pressure and the whims of popular culture. They stand the test of time, and they invite an examination of the concept of authenticity.

AUTHENTICITY

In his book *The Age of Insanity,* John F. Schumaker writes, "Humanistic psychologists have long known that artificiality lies at the heart of anxiety and that a successful cure lies in the restoration of authenticity to people's lives. Yet the radical reliance on competition for purposes of self-marketing has led moderns to package themselves in such a way that any resemblance of an authentic person is disguised beyond recognition. It is not uncommon to hear people referring to themselves, and their abilities and qualities, as a package that is on offer."[66]

When I hear adults discussing the subject of authenticity, especially when I hear individuals express a need to "find themselves" or "discover who they really are," I grow uneasy. This discomfort is not because of the quest itself but rather because so few people who utter these words understand what the quest is really about. Most are simply parroting clichés that have already overridden any chance these individuals might have had for an authentic existence. Who are we indeed?

Every society on this planet uses subtle coercion to pass its culture from one generation to the next. There is nothing unusual or especially mysterious about the process. If culture were not somehow self-perpetuating, there would be no such thing as society. Still, in America, we often behave as if our "rugged individualism" makes us free spirits, immune from outside influence. We tend to view anything that appears to be contrived as being somehow disingenuous. For example, when people in other cultures mourn their dead by wailing in unison, the ceremonial appearance of the display may seem to us to detract from the mourners' sincerity, though surely their grief is no less than ours would be in similar circumstances. Non-contrivance on our part gets dressed up to look like individuality. In other words, it's easy to regard a social device as a contrivance so long as it belongs to a culture other than our own. We prefer to view our own rituals and social norms as ramparts of reality, although, viewed objectively, they may seem equally contrived. This is another act of misrelating that we engage in, precisely because we have not done the intellectual work necessary to live as adults.

In the West, we tend to think of authenticity as the ability to act in accordance with our desires and impulses, while cultural norms act as a braking mechanism to ensure that our pleasurable pursuits do not interfere with those of others. Authenticity must not be confused with nonconformity, however. Authenticity is something that is neither simply defined nor easily achieved.[67] To experience authenticity is largely an ability to see beyond our respective cultures and through our own inarticulate angst, our self-deceptions and illusions, to experience the present as if we actually are here. Now. This is not an ineffable mystical event but rather an instance of straightforward mindfulness.

Most adults in America grew up having similar kinds of schooling as children, the greatest similarity being the passivity of the experience. We sat for hours, days, weeks, semesters, and years with our mouths shut, listening and observing. In most cases, we were forbidden to speak unless called upon, which in time led to a fear that we would say the wrong thing when chosen to answer or read aloud. Eventually, this one-dimensional experience has a strange but predictable effect. It leads to an intellectual apathy wherein we await the next course, the next teacher, and the next expert to continue our docile nonparticipation. But to have any chance of achieving authenticity, we must stay intellectually wide-awake.

Too didactic a culture leaves us cold and renders us incapable of authenticity because we let others think for us. Likewise, too little culture leaves us without the ability to generate the heat necessary for intellectual ignition. By the hundreds of thousands, people in our society complain of burnout in spite of the fact that, in terms of cerebral authenticity, most have never been on fire. For authenticity to emerge, there must be ignition of sufficient energy to amount to fusion. Otherwise the fire will be easily extinguished.

Some very wise philosophers have offered convincing arguments that living an authentic life is more important than having knowledge. The problem is, these advocates were highly educated themselves and so thoughtful that their knowledge shaped the very experience they perceived as authenticity. Living an authentic life depends upon knowledge, but not necessarily the kind we get from formal education. If the postmodernists have taught us anything it is that the popular culture in which we live must be peeled away like layers of an onion before we can have any sense of what genuineness might be.

For millions of Americans, our primary experience for navigating through daily life is steeped in a deep dependence upon authority. True, some reliance on authority is necessary for healthy development. But many of us fail to add the second dimension of experience: independence. By this I mean developing sufficient interest in the subject at hand to construct our own questions and to no longer settle for one-dimensional answers nor tolerate the environment that perpetuates this process. Only if we reach this stage can we move on to the third: integration, which leads us into the kind of consciousness necessary for living our lives as if we are really interested in them. This integration amounts to combining our personal intellectual interest with the external subject matter and then bringing this knowledge to bear in a manner that fuses with our real-life experience, both intellectually and emotionally. This three-dimensional approach

leads to an overarching awareness, or consciousness, through which we become fully engaged in life.

There is something deeply disturbing about people
who become credentialed authorities in a discipline
but never develop enough interest or curiosity to
pose their own questions or read beyond what is
required. In time, authority born of such mediocre
thinking becomes exceedingly hostile to people who
insist on rigorous inquiry. A lack of authenticity is
immediately obvious in people who parrot a party
line but never speak for themselves: the supervisors,
for example, who say what they think the boss wants
to hear but always leave you with the feeling that
they're not telling you what's really on their minds.

As Americans we imagine ourselves sailing our
way through life, making one decision after another
day after day, free of any outside influence and fully
engaged in the dynamics of our own free will. Yet no
other people in any country in the world is so much
the target of implicit messages, both conscious and
subconscious, to act in ways predetermined to
maximize the bottom lines of an endless array of
corporations. Many of the colors we see in man-
made environments are pre-selected for effect. The
products we encounter in stores and shopping malls
are strategically placed so that there are no chance
encounters, except those that are deliberately
arranged to elicit impulse buying.[68] Many of the rep-
resentatives we meet in commercial environments
speak to us using scripts designed to sound both
genuine and spontaneous. Is this for real? Do these
people know who they are? Who we are? Do they
think they are for real and we aren't?

Searching for authenticity is a journey fraught
with landmines and rife with imposters who claim to
know the way. Superficial attempts to seek such

knowledge remind me of the oft-told story of the man looking for his car keys under a streetlight. He admits, when asked, that he didn't lose them there but claims the light is just too good to ignore. To cut through the pretentiousness of popular culture, one must push one's quest for knowledge past the point of strain to the shadows of tradition, and without the aid of the streetlight, in order to re-ask the questions long considered settled. Epistemology, or the understanding of the nature of knowledge and understanding, has to be a built-in component of inquiry in any discipline, in any age, at any time, if we are to move beyond self-delusion. For example, everyone who lived through the 1960s is an expert on that era, but understanding those times wasn't an easy task in 1968. Contemplating the past and recalling our hopes and aspirations for the future with a reflective comparison of what actually transpired is to perspective as a bubble is to a carpenter's level.

When you see a flash of lightning in a storm and count until you hear thunder (which travels five seconds per mile), you can gauge the distance of the storm. Compare this to Immanuel Kant's observation that we are unable to know things in and of themselves. Postmodernism is the clap of thunder more than two centuries after Kant's flash of insight.[69] This doesn't mean our rocket science is not what we think it is, nor that kicking a rock won't hurt your foot.[70] Rather, it's an acknowledgment that the faculties with which we make sense of the world are frail, deceptive, and fraught with existential angst *by design*. Kant concluded, for example, that we simply have no way of comprehending what might be considered Divine knowledge, which means, for all practical purposes, we are incapable of discussing it intelligibly.

Ancient stoics and later philosophers like Søren Kierkegaard and Friedrich Nietzsche, and psychologists Abraham Maslow, Erich Fromm, Erik Erikson, and Ernest Becker have argued forcefully and convincingly that life can best be understood only in its relation to death. Only by facing the ugliness of life and the reality of death can we truly grasp the rapture of being alive, they tell us, and only by embracing the absurd can we experience the sublime. More recent theorists have observed that "normal human thought is distinguished by a robust positive bias."[71] Even so, when these biases are displaced through misfortune or tragedy, the experience affords individuals a clearer and more appreciative sense of the present and the possibilities for the future.

Later life is enriched with little flashes of insight, asked for or not, but only by reaching for perspective are we likely to find it in useful measure. In his novel *The Stranger*, Albert Camus demonstrated that having an imminent appointment with the guillotine presents one with a miraculous sense of mindfulness hitherto hidden but for the whim of focused attention. Less severe but still palpable is the image of Nietzsche living his whole life with illness as his constant companion. I believe a similar analogy can be made when one breaches the walls of cultural pretentiousness where knowledge and education are concerned. Maintaining awareness of the view from outside those walls heightens our experience in life and creates avenues for extraordinary insight.

In our zeal for credentials and with our penchant for misrelating, we've made parallel pathologies out of poverty and illiteracy. This is not a product of anti-intellectualism, but is perhaps over-intellectualism. Who is the inauthentic person—the uneducated, poverty-stricken individual who is barely able to sustain his survival or the well-to-do individual who cannot for his own pretentiousness even acknowledge the other's existence? The idea is to deepen one's appreciation for all experience, not to build a position for passing judgment. Even though knowledge can enable us to live better lives, it does not make us better than other people. The search for knowledge is a virtuous activity, but having knowledge does not by itself make a person virtuous.

Near the middle of the twentieth century, psychologist Gordon Allport coined the term "functional autonomy."[72] He was looking for a way to describe an individual whose internal motivation has changed from extrinsic to intrinsic: from dancing to the tune of others to hearing one's own music. In short, he was looking for people who took the road less traveled for no other reason than that's where they wanted to go. Functional autonomy amounts to having made room for your own opinions and maintaining the personal authority to behave as if you believe them. It is a condition that, by nature, fosters authenticity by setting a stage in which authentic experience is actually possible.[73] In my view, based not on research but on personal experience, functional autonomy and maturity are simply differing descriptions of the same condition. The more authentic we become and the more autonomy we achieve, the better we are equipped to relate to others.[74]

IMMATURITY AND BAD FAITH

It's common knowledge that for any plant to grow to reach maturity it must have all its needs met to thrive or it will in some way remain stunted. The same holds true in the creature kingdom with human beings. As part of the animal world, however, we alone have the capacity to fake maturity by appearing to have reached the state in a physical sense even though we may be light-years away mentally. There are millions of people who try to short-cut the path to maturity by stilling the cultural winds all of us face through a multitude of bizarre belief systems that profess to have the solution to all human problems. The trouble is that such a path is what Jean Paul Sartre called "bad faith."[75] Escape strategies that depend on others to face up to the questions that we should ask ourselves are fundamentally flawed because they increase anxiety even as they appear to comfort. Human beings have a way of knowing and not knowing at the same time. When our beliefs represent bad faith efforts, we fool ourselves only at the conscious level; deep down we deal with our own lack of authenticity through contempt for those who might in any way cast doubt on our sincerity. In contrast, heartfelt authenticity (remember, this actually happens in your head) recognizes itself as such. It's where the autonomy to act independently comes from in the first place.

Authenticity and bad faith solutions seldom exist as black and white distinctions, appearing instead as matters of degree. In large part this phenomenon explains the rift between believers and non-believers, especially in matters that cannot be proven true or false and require acts of faith. The way in which we as individuals manage to cope with our own beliefs and worldviews and remain true to ourselves in our relations with others is a very strong component of maturity. Someday it may prove to have been the most important component of all with respect to the future of humankind.

Wealth is a reality buffer. The gravity of acquisitiveness distorts the way we perceive autonomy and self-creation. Rich people are generally not regarded as being psychologically immature or as being poorly educated; their wealth usually affords them the benefit of the doubt. We overlook the infantile behavior of the very well-to-do, which is great enough in volume to keep the tabloid industry well fed. On the other hand, when our focus is on poor people, we rarely assume that they might indeed be well educated. Moreover, we expect that, given food, shelter, and basic social needs, any educated person will have the capacity to achieve full potential and in fact become a functionally autonomous individual. When poverty strikes suddenly, however, material things once taken for granted assume a role of extreme importance, while social niceties once thought critical evaporate as if they had never existed. The great paradox here is that, when the lower material needs are once again satisfied, only a trace memory of their importance will remain. One's former social concerns will regain their previous levels of importance. All at once, something someone said will again become more important than a good meal. Simply put, immaturity ups the price of existence. To spend one's life spiraling in circles in constant pursuit of things one doesn't need or even want is immature behavior and an exercise in bad faith.

It's incredibly liberating to suddenly reach a point in learning where you fully realize just how little is known, and the earlier in life this happens, the better off you are. The experience is like being freed from a prison cell of one's own creation. Undereducated people, for example, often insist that no one has all the answers, but they don't really believe it. When they learn enough to discover for themselves that it's really true, the revelation comes as a shock. The winds of cultural "shoulds" have blown for so long and so hard that simply staying on one's feet becomes a formidable task. Functional autonomy, or maturity, amounts to reaching a point where the wind is stilled, where you can not only stand your ground but also demonstrate to others that it's possible to stand, and the wind be damned.

The core of anything resembling an education must not so much help us to determine what we want in life as afford us the wisdom to discern what it is we really need. Otherwise, by nature, we will remain stunted and immature. If we don't think these things through, we seesaw above and below the ability to understand anyone who is not considered one of us. In other words, the only way thoughtless people can relate to poor people is to become poor themselves. Above a minimum standard of material goods, true wealth is in large part a condition of one's knowledge and understanding. Eric Hoffer observed that "Poverty when coupled with creativity is usually free of frustration."[76] Surely, then, a component of autonomy in support of maturity and authenticity must somehow lead us to understand the nature of human needs in a way that enables us to bridge the world's chasm of inequality. Leaving bad faith behind, we can begin answering the hard questions for ourselves.

EMPATHY AND REASON

If compassion is a property of life, then empathy must have a role in our exploration of the human predicament. We think of sympathy and empathy as primarily emotional characteristics, but the history of humanity leaves no doubt that these traits must be raised to an intellectual level before much can be gained from discussion about morality. Although we are rigged biologically to value close kin because our survival depends on it, our propensity to overpopulate the earth requires that we stretch the notion of family as a practical way of avoiding conflict.

Degrees of biological relatedness have a formidable effect on the benevolent behavior of lower life forms. When non-human sibling creatures at this level are genetically identical, each treats the others as ends in themselves. They act as if there are no differences between self and other. Indeed, they act as if there is no such thing as the other, as in the case of the insect whose sting to protect the colony will result in its own death. In contrast, for human beings to achieve a regard for others that matches our rhetoric about higher morality depends not on instinct or feelings of kinship but on our willingness to reason our way through the gap that our feelings won't bridge. Cognitive scientist Steven Pinker put it this way: "Love, compassion, and empathy are invisible fibers that connect genes in different bodies. They are the closest we will ever come to feeling someone else's toothache."[77]

Kant argued that rationality is foundational to ethics. Arthur Schopenhauer later made what seemed to be a more compelling case that compassion is the true foundation of ethics.[78] Certainly compassion gives rise to the relatedness we feel with others and thus becomes a basis for deciding how we will act toward them. Still, our relatedness does not yet extend far enough to make compassion in and of itself sufficient to address our global relations with others. I believe Kant was right and that we must reason our way through the issues of distant relatedness. Philosopher Iris Murdoch held the view that "It is an ultimate (and the most important) aspect of human nature, that we sympathize. This cannot be a problem of ethics (as in ought we to empathize?) but is, insofar as can be spoken of at all, something for metaphysics to state, and if not justify, at least clarify."[79] To my mind, such clarification requires a deliberate and thoughtful effort to bridge the gap of our biology.[80]

Thinking through this issue is critical to the sustainability of the global environment. It is our best hope for extending the concept of ethics to close the divide in human relations that allows the people with the top 20 percent of the world's wealth to ignore the plight of the poorest 20 percent. Learning about the world makes it smaller. Learning about people who are great distances away brings them closer. Learning about enemies offers a chance for improving relations. Fully comprehending the forces behind human inequality gives us the capacity to achieve maturity and to help forge the capstone of civilization.

Chapter Three

SEPTEMBER UNIVERSITY

"Education is the best provision for old age."
—Aristotle

"For surely to be wise is the most desirable thing in all the world."
—Cicero

W hen my family moved to Irving, Texas, in the early 1950s, the city was identified as one of the fastest growing areas in America. Life in a thriving Texas community, compared to the small town we'd left in Oklahoma, proved to be something of a culture shock. The pace of everything was faster. In hindsight it seems like a good time to have been a kid. There were clear expectations of right and wrong that ran the breadth of the country in those days. Adults would correct children who were not their own without hesitation. In most cases the children's parents would support those efforts, because it was thought that adults were adults and children were children.

In the early 1950s, the future was thought to be predictable: if you did this, you got that. And yet, looking back from the twenty-first century to that time, it is clear that a large part of what we accepted as common sense in those days amounted to a brand of ignorance whose malignancy ran to the very bedrock of society. Racial bigotry was so prevalent in our community that it might as well have come in the water we drank. People of color were routinely treated with contempt, and acts that openly revealed outright hatred were not uncommon. People who appeared different were suspect. People who questioned power raised eyebrows; people who challenged authority and demanded answers were "communists." Ideas that would be thought of as simply progressive today were then thought subversive at best. During the era known as McCarthyism we had neighbors, a husband and wife, both school teachers, whose views by today's political standards were a little left of center. At the time, however, these two were suspected of being Soviet agents planning to overthrow the Irving school system with a socialistic conspiracy surely in league with the devil.

Irrespective of such attitudes, the '50s are often remembered fondly for their innocence and conformity: steaming casseroles and row after row of nearly identical homes. The dominant feature in the workplace was loyalty, and efforts invested in practically anything deemed worthwhile were expected to pay off. The future that one anticipated could be had but for the investment required. The properties of life were thought to be simple, and above all, stable. Much has changed since then, but there remains an element of our culture readily identifiable for its collective shallowness. It is an indifference that amounts to complacent acceptance of intolerance.

In 1960, at age seventeen, I dropped out of high school and joined the Marine Corps. While in the service I studied for the GED and passed with scores predicting I might do well in college. But, after four years of active duty, I chose work over school. Shortly after being discharged, I became a police officer for the city of Dallas. I'd been told I had an aptitude for learning, but I was at that time a deeply ignorant human being, up to my neck in mainstream indifference. Like millions of others, I had internalized the popular culture of my geographic region, which imbued me with a xenophobic and racist worldview as the one true window on reality. It would be another decade before I embarked on the process of self-education that would enable me to begin awakening intellectually.

Mainstream indifference is a form of ignorance born of inattention and apathy. Depending solely upon appearances, it is fed by pettiness and a gravitation toward whatever seems easiest. It revels in anti-aesthetics, unmindfulness, bad faith, and a total lack of reflection about matters vital for making sense of the world. These are not half-hearted but half-headed efforts. Mainstream indifference is devoid of compassion; it's a hostile, authoritative, and testosterone-laden environment where the weak are ridiculed and the poor are held in contempt regardless of the circumstances for their plight. This anti-intellectual mindset leads to the kind of environment where, as recently as 1998, unthinking white men can assume that it's acceptable to drag a black man behind a pickup truck until he is dead, as happened to 49-year-old James Byrd in Jasper, Texas, or to murder a young man like Matthew Shepard in Wyoming simply because he is gay.

In effect, mainstream indifference is a selfish, cliché-ridden, and narrow-minded refuge for racists, bigots, misanthropes, and misogynists. It's a psychological wasteland where thoughtless people are bound together by a yoke of stupidity that's wholly accepted as plain old common sense. Such thinking frequently betrays itself, however, as seething hatred, complete with public demonstrations of contempt for "others," when actually, a lack of curiosity is the real culprit. The social realm is anti-intellectual to the bone, feeding upon a disdain for eloquence in literature, the arts, and all serious endeavors that require cerebral verve. This deeply internalized conviction is often vested in superstition, intermingled with conspiracy theory, and held so dear that it cannot be acknowledged for what it really is—a profoundly malignant strain of despair shared by a fearful populace who are unified by their own lack of awareness and bonded by a form of hatred so spurious that it feeds off itself. I understand this level of relating because I was a frequent participant before I began my own journey of self-education. I have seen how such insensitivity infects otherwise good people who don't set out in any way to harm others but wind up doing so because of an inherent default to the worst human instincts. Indifference lies at its core.

In 1987, author Elie Wiesel put this mystery of human nature into crystal clear perspective. He said, "The opposite of memory is not forgetfulness. The opposite of memory is indifference. What is the opposite of art? Not ugliness. Indifference. What is the opposite of faith? Not heresy, but indifference. What is the opposite of life? Not death, but indifference to life and death."[81] Indeed, history has shown that indifference is often a breeding ground for evil, allowing social relations to deteriorate to a point where facts are less important than choosing sides. In a democracy dependent on accountable citizenship, indifference is a spiritless sidestepping of responsibility and a serious impediment to achieving authenticity.

My perspective about learning and relating to others stems from the advantage of having had a late start. Even though it's nearly impossible to remember what it's like not to know something after you've learned it, I still have a keen understanding of what it's like to internalize a racist social outlook without the cognizance to know better. Hatred thrives on indifference, but knowledge fosters tolerance, even a measure of tolerance for indifference. I'm quite certain that, had I not begun my lifelong effort at self-education, I would have become a frustrated and anxious individual by now, very likely convinced that any reason there might be for my not achieving more in life was someone else's fault.

Today millions of Americans have such an outlook, and what's so disappointing is that I know how they feel. After more than two decades of voracious reading, writing, and reflecting, however, I'm convinced that curiosity can overpower indifference. I also know that reaching a level of interest about any subject powerful enough to become a self-sustaining form of motivation can be a hard thing to do. Still, I think for most people it's not a question of their having too little time but of how they choose to spend what time they do have. Intellectual maturity is a function of deliberate learning, not of age. True adulthood is not possible without it.

Reflective maturity involves the kind of intellectual honesty that enables clear scrutiny of our hidden prejudices as well as the ability to discern patterns of self-defeating behavior. This need not be an unpleasant experience. Maturity is not the time to shrink from responsibility; it's the time to assume it. Later life is not a time to become set in our ways, but rather a time to figure out how and why we have "ways" at all. It's a time for lifelong liberals to look for value in conservatism and a time for conservatives to do the reverse. Learning in the September of one's life is exhilarating because of the vast perspective that years of lived experience provide. Maturity achieved is an unspoken yet glaring declaration not only that one has lived, but also that one has learned from the experience.

The September of life is all about perspective. The possibility of sifting wisdom from our lived experience is now available to us, if we're willing to accept the challenge and make a commitment to learning and reflection. Enrollment in September University is a last chance for course correction, a final opportunity to experience a life that truly matters as a human being. We should expunge the word *retirement* from common parlance and replace it with *R and R*: reflection and reflexivity. Imagine what a different perspective advanced years would bring to society if, instead of saying we were looking forward to retirement, we said we were eager to begin our years of reflection, eager to sort the truth of our experience from society's fictions. Reflexivity is a turning back into one's experience to retake bearings and reexamine one's coordinates. If the autumn years begin at 50, real education begins in September.

THE QUEST FOR KNOWLEDGE

Our lives as human beings and our relationship with knowledge are wonderfully analogous to the behavior of celestial bodies in the heavens. Like people, stars come in a wide range of sizes and degrees of intensity, as do planets, comets, and even black holes. Stars live long lives through a self-sustaining thermonuclear ignition process. They burn with such high energy that they can provide enough excess light and heat to sustain other bodies in space. Similarly, some human beings continue to shine brightly through one century after another, as their words and deeds add quality to the lives of others, long after their own bodies have been reduced to ashes.

Stars evolve in growth stages as people do. There are small, medium and large stars, giant stars, super giant stars and stars large enough to defy our comprehension of the concept of size. Likewise, human history is rife with examples of people whose accomplishments make them stand out as giants, towering over their countrymen, still offering the light of knowledge and wisdom, just as distant stars continue to light our eyes centuries after the stars themselves have ceased to exist.

People assemble into clusters we call organizations, communities, cities, states, countries, and alliances. Stars form solar systems and cluster into galaxies of every size and shape imaginable. Comets containing unique materials streak through space and provide organic properties that enable the creation of life. Some people likewise seem to traverse life as if smitten by comet dust. They bring such originality and change to bear on society that we use the times of their lives as historical reference points. Black holes, on the other hand, form vacuums in space from which not even light can escape. Throughout history some communities, organizations, belief systems, and nation-states with closed-system ideologies have resembled the physical properties of black holes. When the search for truth must stop because truth is believed to have been found absolutely, imagination and the flames of curiosity are sucked out from all those who dare to get too close.

Individuals, in this analogy, are all born as planets. Some of us are more swathed in comet dust than others; some of us are born so near black holes that ideological escape is virtually impossible. Now, if knowledge is analogous to light and enlightenment, we must remember that planets do not give off light—they only *reflect* light from other sources. Likewise, millions of people around the world spend their whole lives devoid of the fire and fusion necessary to self-ignite and to shine through culture and history in the manner of stars through space.

The challenge for young planets is to move far and wide through the universe without getting locked into an orbit from which there is no escape, and to learn early on how to recognize black holes and avoid them as the sinister forces that they are. Space and human culture are treacherous places to travel without guides who burn of their own volition and not merely from the heat of others. I don't think a planet can teach a planet how to become a star. At a time when so many people are needed in the teaching profession, this notion is very troubling to me, especially since the great teachers we remember for their self-generating enthusiasm are so disappointingly few in number.

Ralph Waldo Emerson suggested that the whole purpose of a teacher is to inspire. In his excellent biography, Robert Richardson described Emerson as a person whose mind was on fire. Sometimes I am convinced that only those whose intellects can be described that way should ever be allowed to teach—and then I'm confounded by the logistics implied. Many young people are distracted from learning by the attraction of celebrities, who are not real stars by any means, and who give off a light not of their own making but generated from the attention itself. How does a small planet get through an expanse of space large enough to gather the material for self-ignition without being caught up and locked into an orbit by a mediocre star or swallowed by an ideological black hole?

The human life form derives its greatest quality of existence through understanding and flashes of comprehension. Although stars in the heavens are very powerful objects, they don't know anything. Humans, on the other hand, can pretend to know something from simply being told about it. But we don't really know anything until our curiosity reaches a level of spontaneous combustion and our own comprehension expands enough to allow us to penetrate the mysteries of life with a deep sense of awareness instead of dumbfounded awe. Without that inner fire, we will be sucked into orbit by any larger attracting body and we will live a planet-like existence, reflecting what others claim are facts; we'll fail to live as self-aware human beings who sense and comprehend the world through our own eyes and of our own volition. Thus, we will die without having reached maturity.

Emerson held that, metaphorically, each of us has the material within to become a star. Absent the heat of a burning desire to learn and understand the intrinsic nature of the world around us, however, we waste that potential. In the field of human knowledge, precious few among us will amount to star status that later generations will recall. Such examples are rare in any given century. Nevertheless, as individuals, we don't have to become giant intellects in order to enjoy a qualitative life and add something of value to the lives of others. We do have to experience self-ignition, however, and our own imaginations have to burn near capacity to have the sort of vitality that inspires others. This is especially true for teachers. We are all born satellites, but to self-ignite and burn brightly enough that others might orbit us, even for a single revolution, requires something far beyond mediocrity.

Let me be clear about this: The key word in education is fusion, and fusion is a property of a mind on fire. Our schools seem to focus too much on instructions for maintaining orbit and too little on finding the courage for exploration. Teachers whose claim to fame rests solely on their ability to regurgitate facts cannot and do not inspire their students to *think*. Self-ignition is a prerequisite for generating enough light to inspire others.

We can probably agree that what one generation wants for the next is the knowledge and ability to live rich, full, intellectually stimulating lives. We hope that through possession of these qualities our offspring will be capable of leaving a legacy that shines even after they are gone. Where the debate begins is in determining how a planet will proceed through space in order to accomplish this feat. At the core of our metaphorical galaxy lie religions and political ideologies, many of which possess deep reservoirs of culture, wisdom and meaning. Unfortunately some of these forces are so powerful that, once one has traveled too close to their gravitational pull, escape is very nearly impossible. Occasionally a planet breaks away and moves about freely for a while only to be caught up in another orbit with an even greater force than before. Many, of course, remain comfortable in their narrow and confining orbits. But, for others, the strength of their attraction causes them to view with contempt anyone not having the wisdom to do as they do. History has recorded these events in an extensive succession of catastrophes.

Anti-intellectualism stems from many complex causes, but one major source is a palpable fear of free inquiry. The overpowering effects of toxic ideologies on unprepared minds make it clear that we have cause for concern. But it should likewise be apparent that our own explorations, driven by a thirst for knowledge and accompanied by a willingness to embrace uncertainty, could give us the strength and ability to light the way to a better world.

The universe is, after all, a very large place, and it seems there should be room for everyone. The problem is that not everyone believes this. Many of those locked into the tightest of orbits would rather see free-spirited explorers destroyed or eternally damned than to be stricken with the pathology of an open mind. How do we create a more hospitable environment where self-ignition is both commonplace and sought after? How do we convince planets that exploration is possible without loss of one's bearing in the cosmos? The only answer I find satisfactory is that we teach these things by example. Nothing else seems to stand the test of time.

MINDS ON FIRE

American educator John Holt was right when he said that "learning is not the product of teaching."[82] And so was Ralph Waldo Emerson, when he said that the only role for a teacher is to inspire. For more than two decades, I've studied any number of subjects with the intensity of a graduate student for the sole purpose of better understanding the world before I have to leave it. While my focus has been on adult learning, I have discovered some very important lessons about the role self-education plays in the lives of children as well. I've learned that uninspired people cannot inspire others about anything. Both children and adults take interest in people who are genuinely interested in something other than themselves.

At the core of my philosophy of self-education is my conviction that an education should be thought of not as something you **get** but as something you **take**. This is not a posture of contempt for traditional education, nor is it an attitude of belligerence toward the teaching profession. What it amounts to, if you really think it through, is a psychological paradigm shift of Emersonian proportions. Thinking of an education as something you take, as naturally as your next breath, is the heart of Emerson's notion of self-reliance. He challenges us today, with even more urgency now than in the nineteenth century, to see with our own eyes, to think with our own minds, and to live as if our lives and our learning really matter.

One would be hard-pressed today to find an educator on the planet who professes to believe John Locke's claim that the mind of a child at birth is nothing more than a blank slate, and yet most educators still behave as if it's quite literally true. Perceiving that an education is something we **get** fosters a passive, stand-and-wait attitude that presumes helplessness unless others come to our aid. Imagining an education as something you **take** gives rise to a dramatic shift in expectations. Internalizing the notion that an education is something you take is the psychological equivalent of taking a fireman's axe to the door of opportunity. It means you don't attend college simply for a degree but rather because of a thirst for knowledge fueled by an internal declaration that you can and will achieve a first-rate learning experience, with or without the aid of an institution. What matters most are your own expectations. Having such an outlook means you are not dependent upon curricula and instead can rely on your own eagerness for learning. It means your textbooks are simply an introduction to subject matter and not a vaccination to inoculate you against the need for further inquiry.

Developing strong interests is the only major force available for the integration of one's knowledge into something that can be characterized as quality of life. Strong interests about any subject can help us master the dissonance we encounter in personal relationships and in global affairs. The world has far too many people whose knowledge remains as compartmentalized as the courses were that parked it there. They live their whole lives with disconnected contradictions that they store in memory but never work out. As a result, they live on borrowed opinions and have to ask authorities the critical questions they ought to be asking and answering for themselves about how to live their lives. Individuals who integrate their learning in an ongoing and sustained effort to better understand the world work out their own solutions. They live beyond the reach of gurus.

The way to help others to internalize the philosophy that an education is something to be taken is to leave a vapor trail of your own interests so visible and powerful that anyone who comes near is caught up in the wake. People who profess to teach and who then demonstrate a lack of enthusiasm for their work project boredom and insincerity. A person who speaks and writes constantly about learning theory without actually engaging in meaningful learning is like a cloud without rain, a flower without bloom, a tree without leaves or fruit.

If you aim to teach, make sure the pilot light is lit in your own mind before you set out to ignite it in others. Yes, it's easy to say that an education is something we should take instead of get, but few people appreciate the profundity of living as if it's true. The joy lies in the truth of this Portuguese proverb: "Live to learn, and you will learn to live."

THE GREAT CONVERSATION

The central ideas at the core of any and all cultures illuminate that which becomes accepted as reality. Religions and politics, tribal alliances, and nationalistic forces define the terrain for those born into their respective domains. It is difficult in many cultures to learn what lies beyond without incurring disapproval. From the time of our birth, the light of our culture shines on what is deemed good, bad, beautiful, ugly, what is valuable and what is valueless. Yet history offers compelling evidence that the people who spend their time exploring the areas that remain dark to their respective cultures are the ones who most often improve life for the rest of humanity. Would we be better off had there been no Plato, Aristotle, Spinoza, Kant, Hegel, Nietzsche, Emerson or Thoreau?[83]

I am persuaded by Aristotle's claim that true happiness must be experienced as a form of contemplation. At the same time, my own study has made me very much aware of the dangers inherent in the pursuit of a philosophy of life. Throughout history there has been no shortage of those who have butchered their countrymen under the guise of truth and justice. Our outrage at these acts has caused us to internalize, at a deeply unconscious level, a mistrust of those who lay claim to higher knowledge. Indeed, the whole notion of an ivory tower in academia implies that knowledge may be used for the satisfaction of a few individuals and not as a mainspring for the betterment of society at large, even though the intentions behind institutions of higher education are noble. It's easy, however, to become myopic in matters concerning education because we habitually assign value to those things that we prefer in life, while we relegate those things that disturb us to convenient levels of abstraction that we no longer need to contemplate.

Fortunately, for those who choose contemplation, academia is not the only path available. Just a few metaphorical degrees above popular culture lies a jet-stream of thought shaped by the geniuses of our species: a legacy of ideas by philosophers, great liter-ature by authors expressing the real meaning of the human condition, and a historical record of how their own actions squared with their theories. This realm is anything but an ivory tower. American scholars Robert Hutchins and Mortimer Adler, editors of the *Great Books* series, called it "the great conversation." It's a realm that's accessible to all who seek it.

If you are poor and lack fine clothing, you can still try on elegant garments in a department store. Similarly, if you can't afford a nice car, you can still sit in one at a dealer's showroom. But, no matter what your situation, if you have a thirst for knowl-edge and are able to read, you can enter the great conversation of humankind. You can try on the ideas of the greatest thinkers who have ever lived, take them home, and keep them with you for as long as you want. The value of these ideas lies not in our ability to call them to memory, but in using them as an introduction to participation in the ongoing dialog. Entering into the great conversation in any manner of one's choosing is an opportunity to escape the default position characterized earlier as mainstream indifference. Moreover, it is the only clear-cut path toward a vista of social and civil maturity.

In Saul Bellow's classic novel *Herzog*, the protagonist, Moses Herzog, is an academic and intellectual who copes with the despair of a complicated life, seemingly unaided by his classic education and his ability to think his way through the problems of ordinary life. Academic scholars often point to this novel as testimony that the philosophies in Herzog's head don't help him with his particular set of problems. While they may be right in a narrow sense, they overlook differences in the way the mind responds to stress when one is ignorant and when one is well educated.

Herzog talks about how "the visions of genius become the canned goods of intellectuals," and how "one of life's hardest jobs, is to make a quick understanding slow." He says, "The readiness to answer all questions is the infallible sign of stupidity," and shows us that knowledge of our own mortality can make us wish to "extend our lives at the expense of others'." Life is life, he observes, "only when it is understood clearly as dying." Herzog tells us that civilized people hate and resent the civilization that makes our lives possible but that "the human intellect is one of the great forces of the universe" which "can't safely remain unused." And finally he reveals that "relief from the pursuit of absolutes" is what makes life pleasurable.[84]

Indeed, what Moses Herzog does, in a deft sleight of hand, is to think his way out of his troubles without being seen as having done so. He has murder on his mind but kills no one. He breaches his existential wall of anxiety with the solace of the very range of his intellect. The story demonstrates that when intellect is used as a refuge, even if—especially if—the reflection appears nonsensical, it is still a relief valve unavailable to the untrained mind.

Unenlightened people don't agonize over differences; they simply set out to obliterate them at all costs. Pedantic scholars fail to recognize knowledge as something other than a possession. Possessed of certain knowledge, they have difficulty imagining what life would be like without it. To be a participant in the great conversation of humankind as a learning and thinking individual is not the same as using knowledge as canned goods for a particular purpose—to justify your own status or position or that of your clan. Partaking in the great conversation is a setting aside of absolutes while you search. By nature, the great conversation is unsettled business supporting the notion that life is a journey and not a destination.

Historian Daniel Boorstin's statement on this topic should be repeated at every available opportunity: "It is not skeptics or explorers but fanatics and ideologues who menace decency and progress. No agnostic ever burned anyone at the stake or tortured a pagan, a heretic or an unbeliever."[85] Pursuit of knowledge isn't the problem. Trouble starts with the assumption that the truth has been found once and for all and that further inquiry is both unnecessary and disrespectful to those in authority. When people adopt closed belief systems that demand rigid adherence to absolutist dogma, then the very existence of nonbelievers fosters contempt at best or hatred at worst.

In the lives of human beings, ideas matter. To be knowledgeable of many great ideas is to increase the size of one's perceptional horizon. It creates a stage big enough for living a meaningful life. It doesn't mean that you can't get precise answers to specific questions or that you can't find the particular knowledge you seek. It means simply that the conversation, by definition, is never over. Ideas that seem to have suffered the deathblow of a knockdown argument have a way of resurfacing with new relevance. Philosopher Immanuel Kant is buried often, but his ideas are very much alive. Among them was the notion that enlightenment and having the courage to think are paths toward maturity.

I don't know what Saul Bellow's intentions were when he wrote *Herzog,* or even if he himself realized the full implications of the actions of his character. The inferences I draw from the novel are responsible not so much for shaping my views as for validating observations from my own life experience. I began a determined effort to become self-educated in my mid-thirties, late enough to retain some memory of the frustration that comes with a worldview internalized from popular culture, with its inherent baggage of geographical bias and ethnocentric prejudices. I'm painfully aware of how ignorance feeds dissatisfaction, and now I am able to contrast that with more than two decades of deeply gratifying study. Bellow and his protagonist Herzog may be completely oblivious to the fact that depth of knowledge offers a release of anxiety through the simple process of reflection, but experience has proved to me that it does. As I see it, a deep reservoir of knowledge about the ways of the world acts much in the same manner as a dissipative structure—it releases angst through a journey of considerations not available to those who lack the knowledge necessary to explore a problem instead of reacting violently to it.

In these times the call for thinking things through deeply is often scoffed at by people who otherwise seem to be intelligent. But hundreds of years ago a Roman philosopher and statesman named Seneca argued that everything in life hinges on our thinking ability. To Seneca, philosophy was a holy enterprise that spawned community and encouraged the enhancement of human relations. In a letter to a friend, he proposed that the custom of beginning a letter with hopes of finding the addressee in good health would better be replaced by saying, "I trust this finds you in the pursuit of wisdom."[86] For Seneca, the great promise that philosophy held for humanity was *counsel*. He argued that only through philosophy can we awaken from culture and that we should accept the premise that "philosophy's power to blunt all of the blows of circumstance is beyond belief."[87]

Given the materialistic nature of the society we live in today, it's not surprising that Seneca's values are shouted down in our marketplace. Still, I find it maddening that so many people with so much apparent natural intelligence have become so duped by popular culture that they don't intuitively comprehend that the great conversation is a quest for quality of life. Living as if this is not so, undermines our ability to make sense of our lives.

Our literature and our real-life dramas portray every conceivable act of courage, honor, injustice and human tragedy. Through their examples we acquire the means to articulate our own responses to life's great questions in terms familiar to our own individual circumstances. Without such experience we are ill-prepared to make the everyday choices that guide our lives. Worse still, when we are fundamentally ignorant about the human condition, we are ripe for political propagandists who would ask us to act against our own interests by blaming others for matters that divert our attention from the real issues. To be intimately aware that others have faced problems greater than our own and to have their examples to draw upon is a beneficial form of exploration and a method for releasing anxiety. To be knowledgeable about the human condition is to be better prepared to deal with it. To understand humanity's existential past offers us an informed awareness on which to base our expectations for the future. To engage oneself in the great conversation is to take on a responsibility that fosters maturity.

ANTI-INTELLECTUALISM

Claims to knowledge tend to come from two primary centers. One type derives from association and the other from reasoning. Experience shows that relationship and association can easily trump intellect in almost any situation.

In claims to truth by association, the logic goes like this: Because my group says this is so, it must be true; and even if it's wrong, "we" are still right. This kind of thinking is especially prevalent during childhood and adolescence. Street gangs live truth by association as a badge of honor.

When we are young, most of us parrot the ideas we hear bandied about by our friends and family. In time, our associations and the ideas we encounter in this way become internalized into an inarticulate worldview composed of wide-ranging ideologies and muddled metaphors, but we resist any suggestion that our opinions might be wrong. It's the fuel and motivation of zealots: "Take issue with what we say, and you take issue with us." In other words, "we"

becomes the operative word. "Our kind" is self-justi-
fying; right or wrong is of lesser importance. We
prove dedication and loyalty to our groups by
attacking the positions of those who are opposed to
"us" regardless of the reason. And thus, young men
enthusiastically demonstrate their willingness to go
to war without any idea, whatsoever, of the reasons
for doing so. On the one hand, this can be thought
of as a noble trait of self-sacrifice, but on the other,
it is precisely the kind of attitude that feeds ideological black holes.

The great misfortune of anti-intellectualism in
American culture is that in so many areas of life the
pursuit of knowledge is shunned in favor of a posture of association. There is indeed a bit of wisdom
in the notion that one cannot know everything, and
it is with this deeply felt but unarticulated awareness that ordinary people, both with and without
college degrees, understand intellectual pretentiousness when they see it. But the fact that we
can't nail reality to the wall in no way means that
ignorant people are in a better position to make
decisions than people who are knowledgeable
about the matters at hand. America's millions of
dysfunctional families are not the way they are
because they know too much about relationships
and human behavior. Try functioning in a foreign
country without learning its language. Try working
in an occupation about which you have no knowledge. Try performing surgery without any familiar-
ity with anatomy.

Anti-intellectualism as a key orientation toward
life is absurd. But still, millions of Americans' sole
inclination toward civic involvement is to shower
contempt and outright hatred on all vestiges of government and everything it represents. Yet these

same individuals won't give a second thought to heralding the U.S.A. in xenophobic fashion as the greatest nation on earth and for what other reason than that it has an inefficient form of government which, in comparison to others, works quite well.

A significant number of the problems we face can be characterized as "us versus them" dichotomies— the great and gaping intellectual fault lines that divide Americans and indeed the peoples around the world, into diametrically opposed ideological camps. After centuries of debate, these intellectual differences reveal themselves still in the clash between the religious person and the atheist over the existence of a deity; between the materialist and the idealist over the essence of life; between the technologist and the Luddite over the value of free markets versus human beings; between the contrasting values of acquisitiveness and generosity, and over the moral dilemma of whether people should be viewed as means or as ends in themselves. Much of this divide takes a form that stills discussion and assumes a posture that is inherently anti-intellectual.

In his book *Anti-Intellectualism in American Life,* Richard Hofstadter said, "To be sure, intellectuals, contrary to the fantasies of cultural vigilantes, are hardly ever subversive of a society as a whole. But intellect is always on the move against something: some oppression, fraud, illusion, dogma, or interest is constantly falling under the scrutiny of the intellectual class and becoming the object of exposure, indignation, or ridicule."[88] Hofstadter warned that "frantic orthodoxy is a method for obscuring doubt," which in part is why literature and learning have been stigmatized as useless by those who would have us act without thinking.[89]

The second kind of claim to knowledge is centered in educated reasoning and in a continuous quest for the better argument. Given a chance to learn, free of the gravity of association, we can develop the autonomy to think as individuals. The veil and power of association will fall away as we become increasingly objective, able to see ourselves and our group as one of many groups, among whom none is necessarily right purely as a result of being who they are. This is the spirit of exploration.

Our outlook on life is a byproduct—or a reward, if you prefer—that derives from our curiosity and from the level of interest we bring to better understanding the world around us. It's not too bold to say that the very act of understanding is itself a creative and supportive defense mechanism that not only enhances the quality of our individual lives but also increases the chances of cultivating our humanity. Life is incredibly complicated—so complicated that we bestow great rewards on those who propose to simplify it. Yet, the more profound and dogmatic these pronouncements of simplification sound, the more serious dunces their advocates become. Popular culture rounds off the mysteries of life far short of qualitative understanding. Custom, as Santayana noted, "does not breed understanding but takes its place."[90] It exacerbates our propensities for nationalism and ethnocentrism. Popular culture attempts to define value for us and thereby short-circuits the thinking required to know value when we see it. In essence, pop culture raises the ante of existential anxiety and gives rise to conspiratorial worldviews, which of necessity make "others" out of our neighbors. Until we acknowledge that matters of the heart really occur and exist only in the head, we are doomed to follow a map with false knowledge as the starting place.

My own personal experience suggests that only
when our individual levels of interest reach critical
mass will we experience the kind of enthusiasm that
others find contagious, transforming the environment to one where people can settle important matters as exercises of reason without falling into
hatred for those who see the world differently. The
geographical nature of belief becomes transparent at
election time, when it's obvious that whole regions of
the country hold views in keeping with the particular wants and needs of their areas. This fact should
render us suspicious of the virtuous objectivity of
our own views and prompt us to engage in the kind
of learning that will enable us to see through it. Only
through deliberate integration of our street smarts
with our objective search for knowledge are we ever
likely to nullify the anti-intellectualism that so readily surfaces during national elections, revealing a rift
among people based primarily on association and
perceptions of status. Would that each man and
woman around the globe were educated to the point
where the better argument mattered more than
association. Then the words maturity and civilization would be interchangeable.

EDUCATION AS UNDERSTANDING

The active pursuit of a liberal education is not a
quest of indulgence in trivial matters but is instead
the most life-centering, life-anchoring thing we can
do. Gaining perspective, learning to push purposeful inquiry past the popular rounding-off point, cul-
tivates a more qualitative existence for individuals
and whole societies. Depending, of course, on good
health, perspective is what we have left when all of
our local concerns fade away. You don't have to

become a writer to anchor your perspective to a force that will conquer the existential anxiety of your human existence, but you do have to *think* if you hope to have any effect at all. If we could figure out how to set aside the contempt educated people have for those below them in the knowledge hierarchy and replace it with a demonstrable enthusiasm for learning, we might reach the necessary understanding to prevent us from drowning ourselves, as Neil Postman once suggested, "in a sea of amusements."[91]

In his book *The Disciplined Mind*, Howard Gardner advocates thinking of education as an understanding developed around three core concepts: truth, beauty, and the notion of good.[92] He suggests, and I wholeheartedly (or perhaps I should say, whole-headedly) agree, that education as deep understanding is appropriate for humanity at large.[93] Gardner, who is perhaps best known for his theory of multiple intelligences, advocates an education for young people based upon gaining a multifaceted understanding of life.[94] He writes, "We need an education that is deeply rooted in two apparently contrasting but actually complementary considerations: what is known about the human condition, in its timeless aspects; and what is known about the pressures, challenges, and opportunities of the contemporary (and coming) scene. Without this double anchoring, we are doomed to an education that is dated, partial, naïve, and inadequate."[95]

Those of us with many years of experience are in the best position to articulate Gardner's concern to the educators in our local communities. Our experience in life, if we really examine it, should make the need for deep understanding self-evident. We can appreciate John Holt's assertion that "figuring out what [we] don't know or aren't sure of is the greatest intellectual skill of all."[96] The only practical way to reform education for younger generations and ensure the nation's mental health is to awaken the older generations and take advantage of what they've learned about living.

Gardner quotes Charles Darwin about fostering early motivation: "It may be more beneficial that a child should follow energetically some pursuit, of however trifling a nature, and thus acquire perseverance, than that he should be turned from it, because of no future advantage to him."[97] Intrinsic motivation has roots in the pleasure of discovery. Look at the problem from the perspective of teenagers. Uninspired teenagers suffer enormous anxiety from being overly defined by others, but teenagers who are deeply interested in almost anything are much less intimidated by what others think of them. The same is true for adults. Indeed, Mihaly Csikszentmihalyi describes the *flow* state as one of intense concentration where time loses its meaning and significance.[98] Flow is a product of deep interest and an exercise of conducting your life as if you are really interested in living. Thus, developing strong interests would seem to be a deeply embedded feature of maturity, but unfortunately too few professional educators seem to make this connection.

It's also useful to think of education as understanding from a strictly biological perspective. Understanding is the very task that the brain spends every second of every day of its life working to achieve. The brain uses all of its waking hours matching patterns with past records, looking for similarity, trying with all its might to understand, trying to keep us from being harmed by unfamiliar circumstances which we are not yet prepared to handle. At night, in rapid eye movement (REM) sleep, the brain reconciles our unfinished emotional business through dreams using the language of metaphor. It also resets its neural patterns for instinctive behavior, and in doing so readies us for a new day.[99] Knowing something about how the brain works affords us extraordinary insights in helping it to help us. Understanding the brain's unrelenting quest to interpret the world for the sake of our own well-being should provide us with the impetus to give it all the tools it needs to do the job.

Acquiring new knowledge lays down new patterns, adding to our repertoire for recognizing similarities in unfamiliarly territory. Moreover, once we understand this biological predisposition for making sense of the world, it's hard to imagine anything more effective in the realization of a civilized planet than the qualitative and quantitative equipping and nourishment of brains on a grand, magnificent, and global scale.

Americans tend to view the world through a prism of values dictated by our livelihoods, our sense of time and place, our geographical bias, and the relational associations that go with them. In other words, we grow up learning to view the world in ways that promote our self-interest and the well-being of ourselves and our kin. In the same manner that celestial bodies bend space and slow time, human beings distort value and bend the power of their respective cultures to their own ends. Socrates knew that sorting out this distortion and developing a deep understanding of ourselves and how we arrive at our conclusions about values is one of life's most rewarding enterprises. Of course, we must see to our own interest in order to survive, but there is great danger in being blinded by "our" own interests. Socrates declared that he was a wise man simply because he was aware of just how little he knew, but his personal pursuit of knowledge was nevertheless unrelenting. If we don't do likewise, then we are doomed to accept spoonfed culture masquerading as truth that's nothing more than a desired reality achieved through association with people who, like ourselves, will benefit from that reality.

The survival of primitive human beings depended in large part on their ability to read the environment as effectively as we now read books. They had to recognize which path was dangerous and which offered opportunity. Contemporary humans require no less knowledge of our cultural environment. The pursuit of education as understanding, in my view, depends upon a robust effort to gain deeper knowledge in matters that affect the quality of our lives: racism, gender bias, generational differences, self-motivation, the aesthetics of art and science. Such reflection is integral to what it means to be educated. The test of life is a qualitative measure of existence, not a letter grade on a report card. Every adult has a philosophy of life, a worldview and an internalized hierarchy of values. But how many of us can explain, if asked, what these are and how we acquired them? Not many, I'm afraid. In far too many cases it may be more appropriate to say we don't have ideas so much as they have us.

Few pursuits are more powerful or more enlightening than discovering the genealogy of our own values. What is important to us and why do we think so? What metaphors construct our valuations of value? What do we think of other cultures and why do we hold these views? In many parts of the world ethnocentric grudges still linger from wars fought centuries ago. Why do people perpetuate hatred for generations when no living person can remember why his or her group hates the other except that hating is accepted as the proper thing to do? What anachronistic behaviors in our society do we accept as proper without knowing why?

Reaching deeper levels of understanding often requires immersing ourselves in arguments that run counter to our own sense of values and our ideas about the nature of reality itself. In the not-too-distant future, our contemporary biases, whatever they may be, will be clearly discernible to someone reading historical texts about us. It is only through deeper understanding that we perceive and appreciate our inconsistencies and that we use this dissonance to make positive changes *today* that will lead to better tomorrows. Any attempt to define moral progress is incomplete without acknowledging our mistakes while we are still in the process of making them.

As noted earlier, human beings are yoked with a sense of anxiety that can't be rid by therapy. It can be ignored or kept at bay by illusion, but we pay a price for that. No matter what we do, think, or believe, we will always feel the pull and tug of this deep-seated anxiety, which at its core is an existential fear of nonexistence. Understanding can ease this fear. In my experience, deeper understanding is a fundamental property of what Mihaly Csikszentmihalyi describes as an autotelic personality.[100] This is a condition wherein understanding and internal motivation are bound together so closely that it's hard to tell where one ends and the other begins.

The self-help movement has exacerbated the anxiety of the human condition, first by portraying unhappiness as a pathology, and second by promoting an inward journey without making sure that some knowledge of consequence is actually present. I suspect this traces in part to a misreading of Plato, who, along with Socrates, argued that the knowledge we require for living a good life already resides within us. Granted, Socratic questioning can pull from us wisdom that we were unaware we possessed, but it's an understanding of the external world in other contexts that enables us to recognize this as knowledge in the first place. That's the tricky part. We understand through the process of having already understood. Even though wisdom seems to spring forth from our lips at the behest of a wise counselor, as if it's originating solely from within, it is knowledge because we have already recognized its value in other circumstances.

Growth comes with learning how to embrace life with an intellectual awareness equal to the task of deriving wisdom from experience, and continuing the pursuit, even when the going gets tough and the understanding elusive. To do this we have to learn to care about more than just what others think. We have to learn to discern value for ourselves. Real self-help does not come from someone else's list of things we should do or believe.

Ideally, self-help teachings would encourage people from all walks of life into a default mode of autotelic behavior. Imagine the expansion in the quality of human life on this planet if ever-increasing numbers of people were to care more about the consequences of their actions than they cared about how well their actions fit with the expectations of society. But how do you convince people of the value of an examined life? Surely asking more of ourselves in maturity is a step in the right direction and one which requires that we probe into issues at the very roots of education.

A thirst for knowledge is for many an acquired taste, and it must build on itself before it becomes a reward in its own right. I know from personal experience that autotelic behavior can be learned. Intrinsic motivation, self-directed inquiry, peak experiences, and flow most definitely are key factors in my own self-education. I've learned to value understanding as an unparalleled advantage, even if the light shed shows me to be in error—especially if such is the case.

All of this Socratic sorting out and examining of one's life used to be considered the Holy Grail in the quest for a liberal education, a goal which at times seems to have been eclipsed by the need to be a "winner," whatever that might mean in the lexicon of popular culture at any given time. It's sad that, even in the heyday of liberal education, strong proponents were often timid in making claims about its practical value.[101] And yet, a liberal education lays the very foundation for understanding what's truly important in life and for seeing everything in a clearer light. Having a better view of reality gives us a context for examining our lives and the ability to define value without worrying ourselves excessively about what others will think.

Naysayers remind us constantly that the aesthetics of art, music, poetry and literature don't help us live in a practical sense, and yet, when pressed, they will admit that these properties give us something to live for. Do they think we are so dim as not to be able to discern that having something to live for is, in and of itself, an aid to living? In *The Substance of Style*, Virginia Postrel tells us that the "aesthetic imperative" is here to stay and that we are hardwired for the sensory pleasure given to us by those things that add beauty to life.[102] She says, "Aesthetic skills are real skills. While not analytical, they nonetheless help us to perceive and understand the world."[103]

What is it in particular about the things we surround ourselves with that makes them seem to matter so much? I believe that a universal characteristic of the artistic works that give us aesthetic pleasure is that at some point in their creation they are the subjects of carefully applied attention. If so, we've only to extend our appreciation for the goods that add quality to our lives out to the people who created them to enhance our understanding of the world and, in turn, to appreciate our goods all the more.

We pay an internal price as individuals for the bliss of ignorance, and society at large pays a price for a citizenry whose search for inner wisdom is pointless because there is so little to be examined. Without an ample understanding of the outer world there *is* no inner world. One provides the context for the other. It's as inconceivable to seek the inner self without the ability to construct and interpret the experience from an outer or larger perspective, as it would be to tour Chicago without having any concept of city.

When viewed together with the properties of life discussed in this book, and with the expectation of gaining valuable knowledge from experience, our inherent human contradictions provide ample context for those of us in the September of life to automatically enroll in September University. While past mistakes may have barred entry to many opportunities in life, this time we get extra credit for our misfortunes.

Biologist Edward O. Wilson has conceived an educational effort for renewing the liberal arts by attempting to merge science and humanities into a coherent synthesis. He proposes that all academic disciplines join with their opposing camps of opinion and make good faith efforts to integrate and unify their knowledge. His term and book title for this process is *Consilience,* which literally means a "jumping together" of knowledge.[104] Wilson thinks such an approach is inevitable, although he is aware of how much resistance the movement will encounter. He writes, "Nothing in science—nothing in life for that matter—makes sense without theory. It is our nature to put all knowledge into context in order to tell a story, and to re-create the world by this means."[105] This process is an apt model for individuals as well, except that I prefer the word maturity to consilience. In my view, the two mean precisely the same thing.

Wilson goes on to suggest, "We are entering a new era of existentialism, not the old absurdist existentialism of Kierkegaard and Sartre giving complete autonomy to the individual, but the concept that only unified learning, universally shared, makes accurate foresight and wise choice possible."[106] I'm not inclined to view Kierkegaard's notion of autonomy as absurdist, but I hope Wilson is right about the promise of learning in the future.

Centuries ago, our ancestors taught their young to read the land underfoot, to read animal tracks as purposeful text to ensure another day. The same impetus is applicable in this century for the signs and symbols we encounter daily. If we do not teach children to deconstruct advertising and to read the underlying appeal of commercials, we leave them vulnerable to primitive impulse and the manipulation of present-day opportunists, some of whom might even be considered predators. Embracing education as understanding is critical to our future because only a small percentage of people in the developed world today are up to the intellectual challenges posed by twenty-first century technology, the ever-changing workplace, the multimedia assault on our senses, and the exponential increase in cross-cultural socialization.

Above all, the quality of our democracy depends upon learned citizens. Thomas Jefferson said it best: "If a nation expects to be ignorant and free in a state of civilization, it expects what never was and never will be." I think he might also have agreed that if we as individuals expect to reach maturity, we have to strive to be free of ignorance, or else we are faced with the same illusion about the cost of civilization and the price of freedom.

We have reached an epoch in which the psychological and sociological complexity of everyday life is ratcheting up with each generation. As each senior generation begins to disengage into a more reflective role, there exists a window of opportunity for leaving a legacy of understanding based on putting the present into a more reasoned perspective. Reaching maturity as a human being requires an integration of knowledge and experience into a coherent framework that enables those who come after us to build on our stories. Otherwise, we have not lived up to the responsibility that comes with the gift of life as a human being.

Chapter Four

ON THINGS THAT MATTER

"Our knowledge is the amassed thought and experience of innumerable minds; our language, our science, our religion, our opinions, our fancies we inherited."
—Ralph Waldo Emerson

S omething about aging moves us intuitively toward that which matters. In recent years, anthropologists and evolutionary psychologists have presented a compelling case that humans have always made good use of their large brains and that modern man has no lock on this development. The difference, of course, is in *how* we use our mental faculties. At some point in our past, we slipped beyond the boundary of immediacy into an ever-increasing world of abstraction. Among our Stone Age ancestors, survival depended upon devoting one's full attention to one's present activities, whatever they were at the moment. Success depended on precise observational skills and the ability to make sense of one's immediate landscape and surroundings. Survival required extraordinary sentinel intelligence just to make it from one year to the next. That we sometimes assume that our ancient ancestors were stupid reflects an enormous gap in what we refer to today as intelligence. Our lives, as complex as they appear in many ways, would likely make us seem dull-witted next to our ancient ancestors. That we live thoroughly immersed in routine abstraction, having lost many of the powers for observing what is directly in front of us, should be very instructive to us as we write the final chapters of our individual lives. Our many years of lived experience offer us a valuable reservoir for reflection and contemplation about what really matters and what doesn't.

In his book *Confessions of a Philosopher,* Bryan Magee puts our dilemma in lucid perspective:

> The world is governed by false values. People in all societies seem anxious to do what they think is the done thing, and are terrified of social disapproval. They set their hearts on getting on in the world, being thought highly of by their fellows, being powerful, acquiring money and possessions, knowing 'important' people. They admire the influential, the rich, the famous, the well-born, the holders of rank and position. But none of these things have any serious relationship to merit: as often as not they are ill-gotten, and nearly always they are partly dependent on chance. None of them will protect a person from serious illness or personal tragedy, let alone from death. And none of them can be taken out of this world. They are not an inherent part of the person himself but are merely external decorations hung on him. They are the tinsel of life, glittering but worthless. The things that really matter in human

beings are things that can matter more than life itself: loving and being loved, devotion to truth, integrity, courage, compassion, and other qualities along entirely different lines. But human beings are all the time sacrificing these true values to the false ones: they compromise themselves to get on, bend the truth to make money, demean themselves before power. In behaving like this they are pouring rubbish over their own heads. If they stopped abasing themselves in this way and started living in accordance with true values, their lives would become incomparably more meaningful, more genuinely satisfying. They would even, to put it at its most superficial, be happier.[107]

Deeper still, alcohol, drugs, promiscuity, and even sports and fanciful beliefs often stand in for the absence of meaning in our lives. In the final analysis, however, what matters always comes to rest in the vicinity of relationships. Whether you are a recluse or a gregarious individual doesn't change the situation. Once we truly appreciate this reality we can begin to understand the psychic investment we incur growing up, wherein we confuse truth and objectivity with the subjectivity of association. Perhaps the most telling way to underscore what truly matters in life is to revisit the property of time and ask whether contemporary society's dependence upon abstraction has fractured the very anchoring mechanism that bonds relationships.

One fact about the human species that stands out through time is our adaptability. The long record of human existence is that of hunter-gatherer societies. Our departure into so much abstraction is a very recent adaptation. It makes perfect sense when you think about it. Our lives today depend so much on our orientation toward the future that we barely make time for the present. And yet, our ancestors were bound to the present and to *each other* in the process. The pace of our daily lives has changed dramatically in the last three centuries. Tradition has given way to popular refinement, and the rituals that once served to bond ourselves to one another and the lands in which we live have been overwritten by an emphasis on market values. People increasingly define who they are by what they have. The result of such detachment is that spiraling sense of apprehension characterized earlier as existential anxiety. Thus, as more and more people who are fretful relate anxiously to others, the more and more bizarre we seem and the more anxious we become.[108]

Every human culture on earth perceives itself as having discovered a method with which to live a useful, purposeful life. Nevertheless, there are a few people in every culture who remain unconvinced that theirs is the right path to follow, and so they set out to find new paths to enlightenment. In this way, human culture evolves through time and place, exploring new ideas through individuals who have a thirst for something more than conventional wisdom. Such efforts have a way of straining relationships while adding something of quality to them at the same time. Relational friction equals drama, and we are fascinated by it. Indeed, this book is in part about writing and editing the final chapters of our lives. Absent our sense of drama, what would we have to say?

Every person in every culture whose life has passed the half-century mark can imagine his or her life as a story containing a beginning, middle, and a rapidly approaching end. Maturity calls upon each person to compose endings that will seed new beginning for others. Life begins and ends with relationships. A world in which our children are valued and cared for ensures a world in which future generations will receive the same kind of attention.

One of the most prominent features of aging is the frequency with which we yield to nostalgia. We begin to take solace in memories from earlier chapters of our lives. Plays, books, movies, and especially music that we associate with former days evoke a wish to lose ourselves in the past. Russian writer Svetlana Boym has said, "Nostalgia is a sentiment of loss and displacement, but it is also a romance with one's own fantasy."[109] And herein lies the peril. We have all known people who seemed to slip away into the past as they grew older, until they finally seemed lost in time. It's not surprising that nostalgia was once thought of as a disease.[110] Too much attention to the past comes at a cost to what's at hand. So, in effect, nostalgia is an artifact of time, place, change, and regret, laden with emotional recollections. Nostalgia tends to override curiosity, as fond memories compete for our attention. In short, focusing on the past enables us to escape the present.

In her 1934 autobiography, *A Backward Glance*, novelist Edith Wharton wrote, "In spite of illness, in spite even of the archenemy sorrow, one *can* remain alive long past the usual date of disintegration if one is unafraid of change, insatiable in intellectual curiosity, interested in big things, and happy in small ways."[111] Indeed, it is astonishing when you think about it that we have memories capable of rereading the best chapters of our lives as we grow older. If we use our memory wisely, with the aid of the properties of creativity and regret, we have our own backward glance capable of making our present deeds worthy of recollection.

SPIRITUALITY

We've already discussed the notion of spirituality as a sum of relating and relationships. Now let me introduce philosopher Robert C. Solomon's definition, which is also the subtitle for his book *Spirituality for the Skeptic: The Thoughtful Love of Life.* By reexamining the life properties of reverence and imagination, and by adding the thoughtful love of life to our notion of spirituality, we have both a head *and* heart approach for bettering human relations. Here we take a giant step toward maturity.

At the end of life, all we have accomplished will reside in the memories of those with whom we have some kind of a connection. And if we could find one key word to summarize the core of humanity's greatest problems, a good candidate, as we have already observed, would be *misrelating.* From the beginning, the dynamics of misrelating have had people around the world at each other's throats.

To put the problem of misrelating into perspective, think of learning as a vertical enterprise and relating as horizontal process. Our mistake is a matter of the horizontal not keeping pace with the vertical. In other words, we become technically astute in specific subject areas while our global relationships suffer the consequences of perpetual misunderstanding. Imagine the acquisition of knowledge as hierarchical: ladders and mountains are metaphors for heightened understanding and awareness. We take numbered courses in ascending order to show that we are climbing, reaching higher levels of comprehension. We earn degrees (again a numeric metaphor) and thereby reach an elevated station in life. In similar fashion, a horizontal study of relationships extends from family to friends and from community to state, to all nations on earth.

When we are young, we set out to master the world of knowledge in myriad disciplines. Unfortunately, we do this without benefit of the wisdom that comes later in life—namely, that no matter what we do on earth, we will be judged and remembered in the end by our relationships with family, friends, co-workers, and others. If our horizontal learning has kept pace with the vertical, these others will include people from all over the world. We will have developed a worldview based on learning and not on popular hearsay or on the ideology that comes with a given profession. Moreover, most of the conflicts we encounter and the wars we fight will be seen, in hindsight, as having been predictable because of the misunderstanding and misrelating that preceded them.

The solution to the problems of relating remains difficult, but it's easier to attempt if we have a plan. My answer is this: Learning about any subject in life, for any reason, should include a horizontal effort to understand how such knowledge extends to human relations on both a local and a global scale. A few years ago, some daring educators would have argued that this was essentially the agenda of a liberal education, but that was before the word liberal became the ultimate pejorative expression in American politics. And it was before the most enthusiastic proponents for a liberal education became wishy-washy about the real value of exploring the world horizontally by beginning with the study of our neighbors and proceeding around the globe. Still, which would be the most effective and efficient method for bettering human relations: the funding and supporting of cross-cultural, citizen-to-citizen studies on an international level or simply bombing each other back into the Stone Age? The cyber-world of the Internet offers astounding possibilities for the former.

The truth is that every discipline we encounter, and everything that matters in science and the arts, can be applied to the level of human relationships on an international scale. Some refer to this dynamic as the humanities. In my view, furthering knowledge in this arena of life is the only way we have any hope of reaching maturity as a society. Thus, the only reasonable path to world peace is to think our way through our global relationships and try, in the face of close-minded ideologies, to persuade others to do likewise.[112]

Relating, of course, has consequences. Ralph Waldo Emerson put it this way:

> All infractions of love and equity in our social relations are speedily punished. They are punished by fear. Whilst I stand in simple relations to my fellow-man, I have no displeasure in meeting him. We meet as water meets water, or as two currents of air mix, with perfect diffusion and interpenetration of nature. But as soon as there is any departure from simplicity and attempt at halfness, or good for me that is not good for him, my neighbor feels the wrong; he shrinks from me as far as I have shrunk from him; his eyes no longer seek mine; there is war between us; there is hate in him and fear in me.[113]

The dynamics at work between individuals also govern our relationships in groups. Evolutionary scientists constantly debate the particulars of altruism, but there is no arguing the point that humans are biologically hardwired for nepotistic altruism.[114] Simply put, we look after those close to us, family first. It's the same adaptation process that enables all species a greater chance of genetic survival by protecting the species itself. This is especially true in times of threat. In this way, threat is a family-maker; it prods individual members to wake up the relational aspects of their species, sometimes consciously, sometimes at an unconscious level.

Some of our nation's most celebrated scientists tell us that humans are threatened today by changes in the global environment.[115] I submit that the only way to solve the problems we face in the future is to think of all humans as one family and to substitute intellect for our biological shortcomings.[116] Only by pushing constantly at the walls of our perception can we reach new levels of comprehension, see ourselves as we really are, and thus minimize our impact on the environment. In other words, since we don't instinctively look after the interests of strangers to afford them our reverence and compassion, we have to make up the difference by thinking our way though distant relationships. You've only to recall Socrates' declaration that he was "citizen of the world" to realize how long thoughtful people have been trying to convince others of the wisdom of using our intelligence to overcome our propensity for misrelating. We already extend our relationships intellectually by identifying personally with our schools, neighborhoods, cities, geographic regions, sports teams, countries, and our nation-states. We do this with enthusiasm when we perceive that it suits our interest. What we need to do for the sake of humanity and the environment is to extend our allegiance to include our species globally. In this way, the path to maturity is also the road to world peace.[117]

So, what is stopping us from extending the notion of human family to include everyone on the planet? Look deeply into this predicament and you will discover a disappointing incongruity. Many people in opposing ideological camps engage in an unrelenting war of rhetoric against those with whom they are in profound agreement where it matters most. If they would drop their defenses and truly listen, they would realize this. For example, religious leaders across a wide spectrum of beliefs all teach and preach brotherly love, even as they offer divergent prescriptions for salvation.[118] Or take Richard Dawkins, a self-described passionate Darwinist and champion of evolutionary theory, who is just as enthusiastic in declaring that he is in no way a Darwinist when it comes to social theory.[119] Better yet, listen to what Charles Darwin himself had to say about relating to others: "As man advances in civilization, and small tribes are united into larger communities, the simplest reason would tell each individual that he ought to extend his social instincts and sympathies to all the members of the same nation, though personally unknown to him. This point being once reached, there is only an artificial barrier to prevent his sympathies extending to the men of all nations and races. If, indeed, such men are separated from him by great differences in appearances or habits, experience unfortunately shows us how long it is, before we look at them as our fellow creatures."[120] This regrettable characteristic of our reaction to appearances was true when

Darwin wrote this in 1874, and unfortunately it remains true today. Still, if lesser creatures can adapt when they need to, maybe we can too.

Describing the nature of slime mold in his book *Emergence*, Steven Johnson writes, "The slime mold spends much of its life as thousands of distinct single-celled units, each moving separately from its other comrades. Under the right conditions, those myriad cells will coalesce again into a single, larger organism, which then begins its leisurely crawl across the garden floor, consuming rotting leaves and wood as it moves about. When the environment is less hospitable, the slime mold acts as a single organism; when the weather turns cooler and the mold enjoys a large food supply 'it' becomes a 'they.' The slime mold oscillates between being a single creature and a swarm."[121] Perhaps as our global environment becomes less hospitable, we can increase our awareness of our predicament species-wide and cooperate at a level equal to or greater than slime.

In the 1970s, Lawrence Kohlberg provided a rudimentary template for moral development that shows in part what must be done to think our way to better human relations. In the simplest terms, there are three distinct levels of moral development. Kohlberg identified them as pre-conventional, conventional, and post-conventional.[122] The pre-conventional is a good-boy, good-girl stage associated with give-get and the punishment and reward behavior we learn as children. The conventional stage is precisely what we should expect it to be from our historical approach in raising children: black and white notions of right and wrong, respect for law and order, obedience to authority, observance of rules, and overt demonstrations of patriotism. The post-conventional stage, which most moral educators suggest only a small percentage of people reach, is the development of a big-picture view of life, coupled with the development of a social conscience and public concern that extends relating horizontally to include everyone in the world.

In the post-conventional stage we make up with intellect the shortcomings of our biology. This is where we put the head and heart metaphors into perspective and reason about emotional issues instead of thinking there is simply nothing we can do when it comes to "matters of the heart." This is where we begin to appreciate the powers of spirituality, reverence, and compassion, and begin acquiring converts to the notions of world peace, the rapture of maturity, and a civilization administered by adults. Moreover, this is where we speak plainly about what Kohlberg's study really suggests: "pre-conventional" parallels childhood, "conventional" equals adolescence, and "post-conventional" represents maturity, meaning that most of the people in the world suffer arrested intellectual development and mistake an adolescent worldview for a mature outlook. Robert Bly once described our predicament as living in a society of half-adults,[123] and John Taylor Gatto has said, "We've become a nation of children." In an article about the negative effects of compulsory schooling, Gatto continues, "Maturity has by now been banished from nearly every aspect of our lives."[124]

Most of the moral development theories being published today concern the raising of children. My message, however, is about moral development among adults as it relates to the concept of maturity. Some people are fortunate enough to have been raised with so much care that they are intuitively generous with their empathy; they do not have to be pushed to extend it to distant others. Some are simply fortunate to have had a wide range of experience with other cultures so that they readily view others empathetically. But, whatever our experience, I'm suggesting that it is the responsibility of adults to bridge the humanitarian gap in such a way as to express the essence of maturity. It is the only rational and conciliatory response to the problems we face, and it requires enough functional autonomy to stand up to people who are dominated by the ethnocentric biases of popular culture.

To reach this stage requires that we learn how to de-center ourselves from our perspective on reality and that we look upon all human beings with Kant's vision, which says people are ends and not means. It is indeed ironic that the very moment we begin to feel like uninvolved observers in life is when we have the clearest perspective. And this aspect of maturity demands that we accept responsibility for the conditions in which we live; it is, after all, a world created in part by our own contributions, regardless of our individual roles. We're accountable not only for our deeds, but also for the injustices which we have witnessed but remained silent about. The winter months of life offer a few last opportunities to speak up before we leave a legacy of indifference.

In the simplest sense, conventional "wisdom" comes with the built-in, self-referring consolation that things are as they seem and that our senses apprehend what is really present, even though empirical study has shown this to be false. The earth appears flat to us, and yet we have learned that it is round. We perceive ourselves as standing still even though the earth is moving at high velocity. The sun appears to revolve around the earth, but we have learned the reverse is true. In similar fashion, millions of people make daily judgments about "other" people, based on what they consider commonsense observations, but which turn out upon examination to be nothing but stereotypical biases. In every avenue of life, learning renders common appearances to be false. Indeed, we are most prone to anger and resentment when our expectations about others are based on misinformation and misinterpretation. In other words, learning in depth about others is a way to develop a more mature outlook and a way to avoid misrelating by dissipating unnecessary anxiety.

The works of many writers, both religious and secular, represent an effort to grasp an ultimate spiritual connection among human beings. Marcelo Gleiser typifies this endeavor in his book *The Prophet and the Astronomer.* He writes, "Time is the absence of perfection. This, to me is what the notion of paradise, with its absence of time, implies; perfection is changeless and thus timeless."[125] Thinking about this quest for a vital kind of oneness reminds me of Plato's theory of Forms, which provided a basis for the contemporary idea of heaven and life after death. While seeming like a grand metaphysical blueprint for symbolic representations, Plato's Forms may instead be simply a property of human perception— an intuitive description of the interior substance of consciousness. The Form is an abstract but ideally perfect template for the inner workings of consciousness. It enables us to make a mind's-eye copy of a tree in the woods, apply it mentally using a pattern of neurons, and then flood our psyche with an image of a tree, thus completing the process of identifying the tree within the context of the imaginary Form. The Form has to exist in our minds already or we can't capture and comprehend the tree.[126]

Plato's conclusion was that the existence of Forms is timeless. Another way to think about spirituality, then, is that we are all connected through consciousness and throughout time (or even its absence). In this way spirituality can represent a profound sense of relatedness best appreciated and demonstrated as a thoughtful love of life and a willingness to regard all our fellow human beings with reverence and compassion.

MATURITY

On the whole, the practice of psychology in the twentieth century has been a grave disappointment. Neuroses seem to have expanded exponentially with the number of practitioners who profess to treat them. Now the twenty-first century is witnessing a call for professional philosophers to enter the mental health fray as counselors no less.[127] You would ask how such a requirement could ever be taken seriously, if we as a nation had not already accepted the idea that only a small percentage of our citizens are expected to think. Are we incapable of comprehending that maturity is a condition from which no adult should be exempt?

In the final analysis, maturity is but an aspiration as each generation deals with the consequences of the immaturity of the previous one. Not to strive for maturity, however, seems to me to be a greater offense than actually being immature. Only by learning and thinking does one become a mature individual. Discovering more about the world is an effective way of coping with the anxiety inherent in the human condition—the process pushes the world back for a more comprehensive view while simultaneously enhancing our ability to function. An emotionally and intellectually integrated effort at making sense of reality is comparable to the bobbing and weaving of a prizefighter to both throw and avoid life's punches—and, in the arena of life, maturity demands a bit of ring savvy. It's a matter of what Jared Diamond has characterized as "dispassionate farsightedness," a willingness to imagine that the self-interest of others interconnects with our own.[128]

We have already observed that at the center of our universe, both literally and metaphorically, lies the profundity of relationships. Mature adults in a grown-up civilization know that all things derive from relationships. Thus, individual responsibility extends globally; our actions as Americans affect citizens in other nations, and it is our duty as citizens to know the nature of these effects. As a nation, we promote global capitalism and free markets as the path for the rest of the world to follow, while often remaining blind and indifferent to the fact that our government's foreign policies foster and support many capital markets that are undemocratic by design. In some cases, the United States even appears to be an accomplice to oppression and partially responsible for the abject poverty of millions of people. Do adults really need to be reminded by terrorists that history, geography and politics are subjects that matter for more than classroom grades?

The concept of maturity appears straightforward at first, and yet the very range of human ability and capacity for experience renders the subject anything but simple. For example, a person can be considered mature in one or several aspects of life and still be quite immature in others. We are all familiar with people who seem to have mastered their career field, but who are sophomores at best when it comes to relationships with members of their own families.

Indeed, one can have a doctorate in psychology and be socially inept.

In his study of human development, Erik Erikson characterized eight stages of life, from infancy to old age.[129] *Infancy* is concerned with basic trust versus mistrust; *early childhood* involves the issue of autonomy versus shame; *play age* brings feelings of initiative versus guilt; and *school age* raises questions of industry versus inferiority. Moving toward maturity, *adolescence* concerns a search for identity versus confusion; *young adulthood* brings intimacy versus isolation; *adulthood* raises the issue of generativity versus stagnation; and finally in *old age* the question becomes one of integrity versus despair.[130] On the surface, the four adult stages seem uncomplicated. We all know people who never seem to have navigated the question of identity; although they are many years past adolescence, they still lack any real sense of self. Similarly, we know people who have been unable to sustain interpersonal relationships at any age, and they remain isolated. Likewise, we know people whose loss of interest precludes any chance of their giving something back to society. And finally, the self-absorbed become easy to spot in old age as their despair preempts their chances for integrity. Simply stated, these people suffer stunted growth. An underlying theme throughout Erikson's work is the assumption that positive connections with other people are critical for personal development.

Longevity researcher George E. Vaillant reminds us in his book *Aging Well*, that Erikson's notion of life stages is only a metaphor and adds two more tasks to Erikson's list. Vaillant inserts career consolidation right after the question of intimacy versus isolation, and he adds the notion of becoming a keeper of the meaning of one's culture after genera-tivity.[131] I think this idea should be taken even fur-ther. Regardless of whether we characterize it as our career, calling, livelihood, lifework, art, hobby, spe-cialty, or major interest, or whether it is simply our job, what we do in life needs to be put into perspec-tive in terms of its contribution. It doesn't matter if we work to live or live to work, or whether the bene-fit of our effort is solely for ourselves or humanity at large. What matters is that we fully understand the value of our efforts in terms of a standard of excel-lence worthy of adulthood, a measurement that lies beyond the simplistic "be a winner" mentality of popular culture. If our efforts have amounted to a payment on the debt of our existence in giving some-thing of value to those who live after us, then we can also be said to have kept the meaning of our culture through our work. The quality of the future is dependent upon good work.[132]

When a massive oak tree or a giant redwood reaches maturity, it offers shelter and support for creatures too numerable to mention. Yet, having reached its maximum strength, it has also become more vulnerable. It offers protection against the wind, but now its size and weight make it more sus-ceptible to damage from storms. The essence we perceive as we look upon the majesty of the great tree is vitality. Its vitality keeps it standing, storm after storm. Vitality characterizes maturity in having a response to the forces that stand in the way of the tree's existence.

All human beings are very similar in this respect. We speak of vitality as an attribute of character. We also use the term "character" to imply a synthesis of our learning and knowledge turned back to meet the world in reply to questions of our identity. We greet the world with a sense of character that says, "This is who I am, and, if you observe my behavior long enough, you will know who I am without asking questions." But, who are we indeed, and where is the vitality that sustains civilization when the vast majority of people in the world are desperately poor, even as they live in the shadows of people of great wealth who, for all practical purposes, pretend the poor do not exist?

Kant argued that living on borrowed opinion is a sign of immaturity and that we do not fully establish character until we begin to cultivate our own sense of the world.[133] Sadly, adult education in recent decades has taken on the guise of basic literacy studies, vocational training or career development. Ideally, it should be advanced study, the kind of inquiry expected of people who are intellectually mature. Scholarship by mature individuals is as important to civilization as clean air and water.

The very essence of the concept of civilization and morality, in my view, stems from maturity and authenticity reaching critical mass. Maturity, in practice, is one generation after another leaving the world a better place than they inherited. Today, the exponential growth of the human population supersedes genetic imperatives in that it is no longer adequate to feel kinship only with those in close proximity to us—family, friends, and countrymen. To have any hope for a sustainable future, we must bridge the genetic divide through intellectual work that leads to everyone on the planet having enough equity to live a decent life without the need to do so at the expense of others.

In every direction we look, we can observe a continuum of life and death: Plants born of seed grow to maturity, produce their own seed, and die. Animals and human beings follow suit. So do stars and even galaxies. The big bang may represent only one phase before the big crunch, which, in turn, could lead to more big bangs and big crunches. Plants and lower orders of animals leave their offspring genetic instructions sufficient to carry on the species. Not so human beings. Our genes influence us much more than we probably realize, but we must also rely on a compendium of external knowledge offset by an internal moral compass—commonly called a conscience—to ensure the survival of future generations. In other words, we learn to care through being cared for, and the nature of our conscience amounts to an internalized barometer of our culture. Thus, the passing on of knowledge from one generation to the next is one of the most important things human beings do.

Erik Erikson's concept of generativity as contrasted with stagnation means the aspiration to bequeath something of lasting value to those who live after us. Generativity is deeply rooted in a life-posture or stance that embraces learning and the property of change. People who desire to give something back to society have either consciously or subconsciously realized that life is a process of flux and fluidity and that to learn is to go with the flow of life. Such people provide the seeds for posterity and the stuff of dreams for future generations. Indeed, those we celebrate as having made the greatest contributions to our culture are not the people who have sought shelter from reality. Rather, they are the ones who have set their sails directly into the chaos of life and its promise of calamity and metamorphosis.

For generations philosophers worldwide have argued over David Hume's assertion that one can't derive an "ought" from an "is." Well, perhaps we can take this notion on faith, but I offer an exception to

Hume: If we are to bring children into the world, we "ought" to strive to make the world a better place. It is most fortunate that maturity arrives as the optimum opportunity to teach from the lived experience of the adult to the inexperience of the young, for without such impulse there would likely be no human race. Care is Erikson's one-word identifier for the life-stage of adulthood. Metaphorically, if not literally, generativity acts as a genetic formula for generational care. It is the seed corn of intellectual posterity.

In this context, it's easy to see why there is so much talk today about a lack of family values. Generativity is only one side of a growth-versus-stagnation continuum, which plays out as care for others versus self-absorption. If the pull toward generativity is great enough, pretentiousness is set aside; external motivation gives way to an inner concern for the future of those who will live on after we are gone. If the pull is toward stagnation, pretentiousness intensifies, external concerns increase, and self-importance drowns any possibility of concern for others. Stagnation in the plant world means there will be no seeds to carry on the order. Stagnation in the human world means that the richest part of life will never be realized and that the fruits of wisdom possible from this cycle of life will not be passed on.

We are all familiar with people who stop learning, who set themselves against change of any kind, people who complain constantly that the world is falling apart because their ability to understand what is going on around them has withered. People on the negative side of generativity fear being swept away by the tides of change. Not only does their rigidity make them uninteresting to be around, but their unrelenting, self-absorbed, inward focus reduces the meaning of their lives to the drawn-out details of their latest surgery. The more they dwell on themselves, the smaller their world becomes.

Interesting people are people who are interested, but people who are self-absorbed are boring. People who stop learning, in effect, stop living. That which ceases to grow begins to decay. Brains that are not used atrophy. Learning, then, is an act of becoming, which makes lifelong learning a realization of being. Immanuel Kant summed up the quest for reason with respect to adults with three questions: What can I know? What ought I to do? What may I hope?[134] In my view, the answer to these questions provides a prescription for maturity. Namely, we should aspire to learn continuously about the nature of knowledge in order that we can make sense of how we are to live.

Those of us who are adults, especially those of us who have entered the September of life and beyond, have one last chance to matter as human beings by clearly demonstrating the kind of interest in life that makes younger generations think we have something going for us after all. We can show respect and enthusiasm toward the properties of time, place, and change. We can use the property of regret with imagination, and use our search for knowledge to resolve our despair and anxiety in ways that move us toward authenticity and generativity. There simply is no better way to deal with existential angst than through a life-affirming willingness to look directly into the abyss. By living our lives as if we are really interested in them, we can be assured of the rapture of maturity and leave the world a better place in the process.

GENERATIONS

For as long as people have been writing about the actions of others, the members of each generation have concluded that the one that preceded them missed the point about what was truly important in life and that the succeeding generation is hell-bent toward the destruction of their way of life. This discord has always been, as the saying goes, more apparent than real. Every generation struggles for something of value; each grows up longing for something they've perceived as missing from their lives. And so, in this way, we are rigged for yearning as a way of coping and adapting through the ages. The interplay of our environment and our biological predispositions confuses us about our character to such a degree that we argue over whether we even have something that can be described as a human nature. Liberal parents have children who seem to be born conservatives and the reverse. Children who grow up poor long for riches; children raised with great wealth often search for meaning beyond materiality.

What has remained constant throughout history is that a large percentage of the population in any given age has, for any number of reasons, remained in various stages of arrested intellectual development, failing by a wide mark to reach whatever capacity they had for broadening the horizons of their thought and experiencing a more qualitative existence. Somehow though, humanity still flourishes, and in many demonstrable ways we are a more moral society than ever before. I dare say, getting a consensus about justice from a random number of citizens on the street today would afford us a better opportunity for fairness than in centuries past. It is simply not possible these days to find Westerners in significant numbers who condone slavery or the many forms of oppression and hostile inequality that stand out in history.

You and I have a decided advantage today because of the perspective our collective experience with learning brings to bear on the future. Armed with many years of life-learning, we are grateful for the Maslows, Piagets, Kohlbergs, and Gilligans who have articulated theories of human achievement and moral development. Even so, when we actually apply our own lived years of experience, we don't need a theoretical model to appreciate the reality that cross-cultural or horizontal learning improves human relations. Moreover, we have enough personal history to know that Mihaly Csikszentmihalyi's state of "flow" and Abraham Maslow's "self-actualization," and Lawrence Kohlberg's "post-conventional" stage of moral development can and should be characterized as properties of maturity, and as such they are an important part of the great conversation of our age. What we have today, perhaps for the first time, is enough objective knowledge about learning to make the first serious global effort to better human relations and therefore experience lives of greater quality—lives that can be said to have really mattered.

As long as we remain living, we still have an opportunity to heighten the quality of the memories others hold of us. In his book *Socrates' Way*, Ronald Gross discusses the Socratic characters who stand out in each of our lives as "carriers of the torch."[135] This is an especially fitting description for the role of grandparents or of any adult in the generative stage of life. Parents often obsess over their children's achievements, but mature grandparents are more likely to put their grandchildren's real interests, and thus their happiness, ahead of their nominal success.

During the decline of the Roman Empire, the great orator Marcus Tullius Cicero wrote a treatise titled *Hortensius*, which elucidates the value of philosophy for ordinary life. The text, which has been lost, was reportedly so powerful that people have continued to talk about it for centuries. The September of life presents each of us with an opportunity to restore Cicero's work. We can aspire to leave a Hortensius behind in any form or methodology we choose. Cicero offered the legacy of a blueprint for the path to moral goodness: developing the ability to make sound judgments, discern cause and effect, exercise self-control over one's passions, and deeply understand our relationships with others so that they might be perpetually enhanced.[136] More than two thousand years later, our descendants, too, are going to need inspiration for exploration and guidelines for good judgment.

The future our children and grandchildren face is simultaneously rich with possibilities and rife with peril: a workplace that toils tirelessly to reinvent itself and a culture driven by a telematic, symbolic cyber-world bent on overriding the autonomy of individuals. The societal transformations ahead due to the dynamics of networking technologies are likely to be profound and continuously unrelenting. Our offspring in the middle and late twenty-first century will need an extraordinary sense of self to embrace so much potential and so much uncertainty. In short, they will need to be much more open to learning than their grandparents' generation. If we as parents and grandparents can know that much about the future, we can help.

Learning and the residual knowledge it provides give human beings a refuge of inner experience with which to cushion the blows of the external world.

The greater our individual depths of learning, the better we are able to cope with anxiety and adversity, and the better we are able to comprehend the dysfunctional nature of bigotry and prejudice. Comparative reflection moderates our feelings about people we have come to view as "others." When we understand something about the character and motivations of people of dissimilar cultures, we are better able to perceive that they have the same needs as we do. Our children and grandchildren are going to live in a world more multicultural than earlier generations ever dreamed of. They are going to have to be better at getting along with others than we ever were. A part of our generativity and our legacy involves helping them prepare for this future.

One night recently, I suddenly awoke with the answer to a question I'd long been sleeping on: What if today, past 60, I had an opportunity to slip through a fissure in time, only for a moment, to advise the person I was at 30? What if, in a twist on Nietzsche's Eternal Return, my younger self had a chance to make a fresh start, to do things differently than the first time? Knowing that the quality of the future was at stake, what would I say? My response in a nutshell came to this:

Nothing important about the world can be assumed from appearances. Nothing is as it seems. Not the history, not the politics, not the religion, not the relationships, and certainly not your worldview. If you believe that only your daily observations and the inferences you make from popular culture are ramparts of reality, you are not only mistaken but seriously deluded. Moreover, you and your society will pay a moral tax for your indifference, excised through needless anxiety and an ever-present potential for misrelating on a global scale.

My additional 30 years of experience have taught me that appearances are profoundly deceiving. Were that not the case, there would be no reason, whatsoever, to assume a need for what we call higher education. Thirty years ago, when I was most adamant in my opinions about the world, my knowledge amounted to little more than borrowed opinion and truth by association. Today, I'm in no position to declare that I finally, once and for all, have determined the nature of things, only that the way to gain ground in better understanding the world is to ask questions every step of the way. Henry David Thoreau was of this mind when he said he wanted 'to live deep and suck out the marrow of life.'[137] But in order to get to the marrow you must look above, beneath, behind, and beyond the vistas of popular culture, regardless of where you live in the world and whose flag you salute. Learn to the best of your ability, all the rest of your days, and you may experience a life rich with rapturous insights.

A LEGACY FOR GRANDCHILDREN

What we leave behind in words and deeds will reside for a time in the memories of those who live on. If we've achieved maturity, the relationships we established will act as seeds for improving interactions among the living. When, by living example, we sanction our heirs to learn the greatest lessons of their lives, we give them something that money cannot buy. We give them vitality and the foundational principle of what later in life comes to be known as confidence. The role grandparents can play in helping their grandchildren develop a thirst for knowledge and an enthusiasm for learning is profoundly important, but it sounds far simpler than it is. Here is a good start:

- Try to remember what it's like not to know.
- Never forget that people who are not learners cannot inspire others to be what they themselves are not. Children see through such pretensions.
- Make sure that you take time for your grandchildren's questions when no one else does—especially when no one else does. Keep in mind there are no stupid questions, only stupid answers.
- Recognize that some learning is painful and that significant emotional events are often great pivotal moments in life.
- Never forget that life's greatest lessons stem from mistakes. Fear of making mistakes is a crippling condition that essentially amounts to fear of life itself.
- Keep in mind always that learning *is* and should be exciting. Enthusiasm is a great teacher.
- Make it your long-term goal to convince your grandchildren, through your own actions, that America's greatest treasures are found not in our shopping malls but in our libraries.
- Realize that every discipline representing a vertical hierarchy of knowledge results in horizontal consequences for other people; the more dynamic the knowledge, the greater the effects. Thus, maturity requires that the horizontal keep pace with the vertical.
- Remember that learning is its own reward. When you help your grandchildren appreciate this notion, you help them avoid internalizing the belief that learning is behaving, and you give them an essential tool for establishing a sense of self: the ability to think for themselves. Having that ability leads to the greatest means of independence a person can have: the ability to define value for oneself, which provides the foundation for autonomy.

With these as your guiding principles, you will be able to encourage a healthy attitude toward learning in children from an early age. As they progress, look for opportunities to broaden their thinking and support their autonomy. For example:

- Help them to discover that the best way to begin to study any subject is to bring it into perspective through their own questions.
- Help them to discover that understanding history enables us to fashion a better future.
- Help them learn to think of knowledge not as a possession, but as a process in which we plot our course in life. Continuous learning strengthens our ability to navigate our way through everyday experience.
- Help them to understand that books are but perspectives; the more books they read, the larger their own perspective will become.
- Help them to understand that we naturally learn more about what we care about, and that a shortcut to knowledge can be found in learning to care.
- Help them to understand that it's easier to become great at what you are naturally good at than good at what you seem to have little or no aptitude for. In other words, building on strengths is a shortcut to confidence.
- Help them to discover that technology is the way that you leverage your skills and strengths. The technologies they grow up with, even cutting-edge computer technology, will seem as natural to them in a few years as radio and television do to us. If you fear technology yourself, do not voice your apprehensions. On the contrary, learn with your grandchildren, with their help. Join in, and benefit from their enthusiasm and natural curiosity.

- Help them to understand that the properties of life discussed in this text represent but a few of the possible vantage points from which to examine the things we most often take for granted. Encourage them to create their own list of properties and to appreciate how they are avenues of insight into the human predicament.
- Help them learn to identify the many guises of anti-intellectualism and to understand it as a tool of misanthropes, disingenuous politicians, and ignorant people. Help them see that anti-intellectualism is anathema to human growth and an obstacle to experiencing quality of life.
- Help them to understand that money is not the ultimate valuation of value in our society, even though most people behave as if it's true.
- Help them to recognize the senselessness of confusing their identity with brand-name products.
- Help them to understand that pretentiousness is not only a characteristic of immature behavior, but also one of life's greatest detractors from authenticity.
- Help them to discover the wisdom in the metaphor that life is a journey, not a destination.
- Help them to understand the language of metaphors and how these imaginings color our sense of reality and shape our spatial sense of the world. In matters of the heart, for instance, reasoning in the head is always necessary.
- Help them to understand Howard Gardner's theory of multiple intelligences and specifically how it applies to their own individual talents.
- Help them to understand that mastering the ability to read not only will open the whole world to them, but also will become its own reward as a relief valve for dissipating the kind of anxiety

that thrives in societal ignorance.

- Help them learn to value and appreciate the strengths and power available to those with the courage to be different.
- Help them to discover how creativity is both a means of distinguishing ourselves from others as well as a subtle attempt at endearment.
- Help them to appreciate Mihaly Csikszentmihalyi's concept of *flow* and the value of learning with optimal effort. We learn best when the challenge is not overwhelming but is sufficient to hold our sustained interest.
- Help them to understand that there is an enormous difference between simply being too distracted by external stimuli to be truly aware of the present moment and being so engaged and enthralled by what you are doing that the notion of time disappears altogether.
- Help them internalize the notion that an education is not something you get, but is something you take. Explain that this is not a posture of arrogance, but a declaration of self-reliance.
- Help them to discover that institutions can be good places for learning, but if your desire to learn is strong and you are interested in the great questions confronting our species, then they may actually obstruct your learning. The way to prevent this is not to let your curiosity be overridden by their curricula.
- Help them to understand that the greatest defense against peer pressure is often found in the courage to be different and that until leaders reveal who they are through their acts of independence people don't recognize them as leaders.
- Help them to understand that there is truth in the old saying that actions speak louder than

words: that the world is rife with people who don't walk their talk, a fact which doesn't by itself impugn their veracity but should, as Nietzsche suggested, arouse suspicion.

- Help them to discover the need to be wary of groups and organizations that discourage questions. Explain the dangers of ideological black holes.

- Regardless of their religious affiliation or lack of one, help them to comprehend the notion of spirituality as a means of relating and as an expression of a thoughtful love of life.

- Help them to understand the dynamics of human relationships, that the success of humanity requires thinking of ourselves as one planet, one people, one family, and that this process requires vigorous intellectual effort to overcome our biological predisposition for kin.

- Help them to understand that generational differences can be understood with effort and that, when you strip away custom and tradition, all people have the same human needs and wants.

- Help them to understand that the differences among us appear far more mysterious than need be. A key to better understanding them can be found in the straightforward observation that people learn to long for what they grow up without. The property of reverence thus applied can help bridge understanding among groups.

- Help them to understand that democracy is dependent upon an educated populace, and its very quality requires that citizens stand taller than consumers.

- And finally—not through your words, but through your actions—help them to realize that there is nothing to fear as one gets increasingly closer to the end of life. This emblazons an image in the minds of young people of the dignity of old age.

A primary goal for the learning of those who live after us is that they develop enough enthusiasm for life to be able to sustain themselves as far as possible above the world of clichés and slogans. Understanding that people believe as they perceive, we might regard anxiety as a form of ignorance and thus create fertile ground for inquiry. If we are to change minds, we must change perception, and this requires active exploration. This is by no means an easy task, and at times the peer pressure and fast pace of the lives of young people make it seem very impracticable. Further, we must consider John Holt's observation that "99 percent of the time, teaching that has not been asked for will not result in learning, but will impede learning."[138] Nevertheless, by focusing on the needs of the generations that follow and working to change their perception, we have an opportunity to embrace Erikson's final stage of life in pursuit of integrity while simultaneously relieving ourselves of the anxiety of aging. Using my own grandparents as a guide, I propose that it is the responsibility of grandparents to leave indelible memories as to just what grandparents are supposed to be like. In this way, the notion that successive generations can lay the foundation on which their heirs will build their lives becomes quite literally true.

Genuine confidence connects at a deep level to the umbilical cord of our emotions; our head and heart metaphors for apprehending the world lead us to the development of a grown-up conscience. Part of the strength required for believing one has a chance in life is bound to the kind of care one has received as a youngster. Grandparents who leave such a legacy to their grandchildren give them something far more valuable than money. Without ever mentioning it, they teach them how to be grandparents, and therein lies the rapture of maturity. The late Neil Postman's immortal declaration, "Children are the living messages we send to a time we will not see," is a lasting aspiration of maturity and a reverberation of rapture.[139]

The caterpillar is condemned to crawl, but the butterfly has the potential to soar above with an all-inclusive view of the world. As humans we complete our caterpillar stage when we reach mature physical growth. If we are to soar like the butterflies, we must do so through the development of our minds. The enhanced view is always worth the effort. Indeed, the very thing that determines the quality of the later seasons of life is the degree to which we are interested in learning more about the world. Our final stage of human development includes the capacity for rapture as our desire to better understand the world helps to make it a better place for those who live on after us. Our moral concerns shift from the behavior of individuals to global relations and humanity's future. If our efforts bear enough fruit, perhaps we will be remembered as wise. We will have left a lasting legacy, and we will have taken our leave with integrity.

NOTES

INTRODUCTION

1. Ernest Becker, *The Denial of Death* (New York: The Free Press, 1973), 55. Becker takes this idea even further, claiming that what we are really trying to achieve is a persona capable of hiding our fear and insecurities about the world.

2. No doubt, many of these activities offer a heightened sense of awareness, and as such they may be experienced as being intensely meaningful. But when you put them into context with a life that matters and the responsibility that goes with it, the meaning often evaporates and these daring events appear misguided and irresponsible. You've only to ask the few daredevils who reach old age for some perspective on their younger days to judge the truth of the matter.

3. Harold S. Kushner, *Living a Life That Matters* (New York: Alfred A. Knopf, 2001), 146.

4. Ibid., 6.

5. Ernest Becker, *The Denial of Death* (New York: The Free Press, 1973), 48-49.

6. Randall Collins, *The Sociology of Philosophies* (Cambridge, MA: Belknap Press of Harvard Univ. Press, 1998), 19. Collins offers a workable definition of an intellectual: "Intellectuals are people who produce decontextualized ideas. These ideas are meant to be true or significant apart from any locality, and apart from anyone concretely putting them in practice."

CHAPTER ONE

7. Bryan Magee, *Confessions of a Philosopher* (New York: Random House, 1997), 441.

8. American commercial demographics are increasingly based on zip codes.

9. Alan Watts, *The Wisdom of Insecurity* (New York: Vintage Books, 1951), 43.

10. Janet Landman, *Regret* (New York: Oxford Univ. Press, 1993). I highly recommend this work in understanding the dynamics at play in the property of regret.

11. Ibid., 263.

12. This point will be examined in greater detail as an ongoing effort to reduce confusion over the expression of head versus heart metaphors.

13. Janet Landman, *Regret* (New York: Oxford Univ. Press, 1993), 40. Landman characterizes regret as being the opposite of cognitive dissonance, "a failure to rationalize or justify one's prior behavior or decision through cognitive maneuvers that may be conscious or unconscious."

14. Ibid., 74.

15. Milan Kundera, *Ignorance* (New York: HarperCollins, 2000), 76.

16. Eric Hoffer, *The True Believer* (New York: Harper & Row, 1951), 91.

17. There is a school of thought that suggests truth is more reliable from reaction than from deliberation. I'm somewhat sympathetic with this view, but I have also concluded that developing such reactions requires a great deal of self-knowledge, which itself requires reflection.

18. Susan Neiman, *Evil in Modern Thought* (Princeton, NJ: Princeton Univ. Press, 2002), 75.

19. Aristotle, "On Poetics," trans. Ingram Bywater, in *Great Books of the Western World*, Vol. 42 (Chicago: Encyclopedia Britannica, 1952), 681-689.

20. Iris Murdoch, *Metaphysics as a Guide to Morals* (New York: Viking Penguin, 1992), 93. Murdoch claims that, in the Aristotelian sense of the term, Auschwitz was not a tragedy. She says the concept of tragedy is obscure. No doubt about it, the deeds in themselves may not be tragic, but to those who live on afterwards their effects certainly are.

21. Matthew Miller, *The 2 Percent Solution* (New York: Public Affairs, 2003), 71. On capitalism's place with regard to luck, Miller writes, "Try too hard to wipe out the inequities spawned by luck and you banish luck's social benefits and

go the road of communism. Harness a healthy balanced awe for luck, however, and you expand the bounds of empathy in ways that make universal health coverage and great schools for poor children a national imperative."

22. Daniel C. Dennett, *Darwin's Dangerous Idea* (New York: Simon & Schuster, 1995), 517.

23. Alan Watts, *The Wisdom of Insecurity* (New York: Vintage Books, 1951), 34.

24. Mihaly Csikszentmihalyi, *Flow* (New York: Harper & Row, 1990), 10.

25. Ibid., 19.

26. Ibid., 21.

27. Ibid., 21.

28. Ibid. No one explains the process of optimal learning better than Mihaly Csikszentmihalyi.

29. It is common for writers and artists to discount the attention given to their work or to deny a social motivation, but few would maintain enthusiasm for their efforts if no one ever looked at their art or read their words.

30. Paul Woodruff, *Reverence* (New York: Oxford Univ. Press, 2001), 3.

31. Ibid., 5.

32. Ibid., 8.

33. Ibid., 13.

34. Ibid., 15.

35. Ken Dychtwald, *Age Power* (New York: Tarcher/Putnam, 1999), 225.

36. Thomas Merton is said to have spoken these words at a meeting of the Parliament of World Religions.

37. Joseph Goldstein, *One Dharma* (New York: HarperCollins, 2002).

38. Carl Sagan, *Contact* (New York: Doubleday, 1997).

39. Viktor Frankl, *Man's Search for Meaning* (New York: Pocket Books, 1984), 86.

40. Ibid., 131-132.

CHAPTER TWO

41. M. Scott Peck, *Further Along the Road Less Traveled* (New York: Touchstone Books, 1998).

42. Joe Griffin and Ivan Tyrrell, *Human Givens* (United

Kingdom: Human Givens Publishing, 2003). This book provides the best explanation I've ever found about the psychological consequences of conflicting information and beliefs.

43. Friedrich Nietzsche, *Beyond Good and Evil,* ed. and trans. R. J. Hollindale (New York: Penguin Books, 1973), 91.

44. Janet Landman, *Regret* (New York: Oxford Univ. Press, 1993), 173.

45. Søren Kierkegaard, *The Sickness Unto Death,* ed. and trans. Howard V. Hong and Edna H. Hong (Princeton, NJ: Princeton Univ. Press, 1980), 22-60.

46. Ibid., 13.

47. Roderick, Rick, *Philosophy and Human Values* (Kearneysville, WV: The Teaching Company, 1991), audiocassette.

48. William Greider, *The Soul of Capitalism* (New York: Simon & Schuster, 2003), 10.

49. Philip E. Slater, *The Pursuit of Loneliness* (Boston, MA: Beacon Press, 1990), 79.

50. Roderick, Rick, *Philosophy and Human Values* (Kearneysville, WV: The Teaching Company, 1991), audio-cassette. Sometimes I get the feeling that in his book *The Sickness Unto Death,* Kierkegaard is toying with the reader.

51. William F. Allman, *The Stone Age Present* (New York: Simon & Schuster, 1994), 247. Allman says, "[The] modern human brain has been designed by evolution for a social life that is not very different from that of the Cro-Magnon who lived in Europe some 30,000 years ago." So, it would seem to me our current way of life is in need of some adjustments that may not seem intuitive.

52. Derek Parfit, *Reasons and Persons* (New York: Oxford Univ. Press, 1984). This book is full of well-documented examples of self-defeating behavior.

53. Jeff Schmidt, *Disciplined Minds* (Lanham, MD: Rowman & Littlefield, 2000), 11.

54. Joe Griffin and Ivan Tyrrell, *Human Givens* (United Kingdom: Human Givens Publishing, 2003), 234.

55. George Lakoff and Mark Johnson, *Metaphors We Live By* (Chicago, IL: Univ. of Chicago Press, 1980).

56. George Lakoff and Mark Johnson, *Philosophy in the Flesh* (New York: Basic Books, 1999), 50.

57. George Lakoff and Mark Johnson, *Metaphors We Live By* (Chicago, IL: Univ. of Chicago Press, 1980), 103.

58. Ibid., 5.

59. This kind of inductive reasoning, or reasoning beneath consciousness, provides the very foundation for mysticism.

60. There is much in postmodernism, post-structuralism, deconstruction, new-historicism, and multicultural perspective that I find exciting and insightful, but the overall impact of the movement appears to be that of an extraordinary opportunity missed. Although the concept of deconstruction had great potential, its application has lost direction and degenerated into silliness. For a time it was (and in some instances still is) chic to claim that you don't know what postmodernism means. This would have been an ideal time to recognize just how sloppy our thinking has become in myriad disciplines and how a lack of critical thinking has produced such nonsensical outcomes as the patronage of astrological gurus and the rise of unscrupulous individuals who pretend to communicate with the dead. With care, postmodernism could have sounded the alarm for critical thinking as a method long past due, appropriate across the board and in every subject that adds meaning to life. There is still time, however. Someday postmodernism might be acknowledged as the point at which we awakened and began to use our gray matter in a manner that honors our existence.

61. Morris Berman, *The Twilight of American Culture* (New York: W.W. Norton, 2000), 178.

62. Jared Diamond, *Guns, Germs, and Steel* (New York: W.W. Norton, 1997), 19.

63. This is not to suggest that laziness does not exist among primitive cultures. Clearly such is not the case. But my reading of anthropology indicates that the meaning derived from the activities that keep hunter-gather societies alive cannot be compared to that of busy work in an industrial setting.

64. David Riesman, *The Lonely Crowd* (New Haven, CT: Yale Univ. Press, 2001).

65. George Bernard Shaw, *Man and Superman* (New York: Brentano's, 1903), xxxi-xxxii.

66. John F. Schumaker, *The Age of Insanity* (Westport, CT: Praeger, 2001), 73.
67. So far, the best way I've found to define authenticity is to point to the times when I'm sure of what it's not.
68. If this were not bad enough, advertisers are increasingly resorting to what is called "stealth" marketing, setting up artificial encounters through the use of actors so that what appears to be a spontaneous and chance meeting is nothing more that a contrived method of introducing new products.
69. Certainly to do justice to this storm metaphor, many other thinkers ought to be included as having contributed to the thunder, but the only one who cannot be overlooked, in my view, is Frederich Nietzsche.
70. Kant's notion of "things in themselves" has been assaulted by too many philosophers to mention, but it has never, to my mind, been satisfactorily refuted.
71. Shelley E. Taylor, *Positive Illusions* (New York: Basic Books, 1989), 7.
72. Gordon W. Allport, *The Person in Psychology* (Boston, MA: Beacon Press, 1968), 79.
73. Gordon W. Allport, *Becoming* (New Haven, CT: Yale Univ. Press, 1955), 79. As early as 1955, Allport asserted that the whole enterprise of existentialism was in need of a blood transfusion, so that dealing with anxiety might be put in a more humanistic perspective. Yet here we are in the twenty-first century still awaiting the infusion of that wisdom.
74. Edward L. Deci and Richard Flaste, *Why We Do What We Do* (New York: Penguin Books, 1995), 6.
75. Jean Paul Sartre, *Being and Nothingness*, trans. Hazel E. Barnes (New York: Washington Square Press, 1993), 86-112.
76. Eric Hoffer, *The True Believer* (New York: Harper & Row, 1951), 34.
77. Steven Pinker, *How the Mind Works* (New York: W.W. Norton, 1997), 401.
78. Bryan Magee, *Confessions of a Philosopher* (New York: Random House, 1997), 397.
79. Iris Murdoch, *Metaphysics as a Guide to Morals* (New York: Viking Penguin, 1992), 64.

80. Steven Pinker, *The Blank Slate* (New York: Viking, 2002), 305. As an aside to the question of whether there is something that can be called human nature Pinker writes, "Every student of political science is taught that political ideologies are based on theories of human nature. Why must they be based on theories that are three hundred years out of date?" Why indeed? How can we hope to improve political relations among the countries of the world if the very discipline we study as a means is itself hopelessly immature?

CHAPTER THREE

81. Diane Hirth, "Wiesel Warns of Indifference," Fort Lauderdale *Sun Sentinel*, May 8, 1987.

82. John Holt, *Learning All the Time* (Reading, MA: Perseus Books, 1989), 160.

83. No doubt there are scores of scholars who would not only point out the arbitrariness of my list but make a case to the contrary. Still, the works of these individuals, whether one agrees with them or not, are worthy of serious reflection.

84. Saul Bellow, *Herzog* (New York: Penguin Books, 1961), 74, 139, 155, 162, 182, 304, 311, 323.

85. Daniel J. Boorstin, "The Amateur Spirit," in *Living Philosophies,* ed. Clifton Fadiman (New York: Doubleday, 1990), 24.

86. Seneca, *Seneca: Letters from a Stoic,* ed. and trans. Robin Campbell (New York: Penguin Books, 1969), 60.

87. Ibid., 103.

88. Richard Hofstadter, *Anti-Intellectualism in American Life* (New York: Vintage Books, 1962), 45.

89. Ibid., 123.

90. George Santayana, *Skepticism and Animal Faith* (New York: Dover, 1923), 6.

91. Neil Postman, *Amusing Ourselves to Death* (New York: Viking Penguin, 1985), vii.

92. Howard Gardner, *The Disciplined Mind* (New York: Simon & Schuster, 1999), 16.

93. Ibid., 224.

94. Howard Gardner, *Frames of Mind* (New York: Basic Books, 1993). Gardner suggests there are seven different types of

intelligence: mathematical, linguistic, musical, spatial, kinesthetic, interpersonal, and intrapersonal.

95. Howard Gardner, *The Disciplined Mind* (New York: Simon & Schuster, 1999), 20.

96. John Holt, *Learning All the Time* (Reading, PA: Perseus Books, 1989), 20.

97. Howard Gardner, *The Disciplined Mind* (New York: Simon & Schuster, 1999), 76.

98. Mihaly Csikszentmihalyi, *Flow* (New York: Harper & Row, 1990). This book is on my short list of the best self-help books of the past quarter century. Understanding the concept of flow is central to the development of self-knowledge.

99. Joe Griffin and Ivan Tyrrell, *Human Givens* (United Kingdom: Human Givens Publishing, 2003). The book does indeed live up to the description in its subtitle: *A New Approach to Emotional Health and Clear Thinking.*

100. Paolo Inghilleri, *From Subjective Experience to Cultural Change*, trans. Eleonora Bartoli (New York: Cambridge Univ. Press, 1999), 92.

101. In his book *Why Education Is Useless* (Philadelphia, PA: Univ. of Pennsylvania Press, 2003), Daniel Cottom takes on the anti-intellectual establishment by making their arguments better than the anti-intellectuals themselves are capable of making them. Then he ups the ante of discourse by making the case that because education may be considered useless certainly doesn't mean it's valueless.

102. Virginia Postrel, *The Substance of Style* (New York: HarperCollins, 2003), 164.

103. Ibid., 170.

104. Edward O. Wilson, *Consilience* (New York: Alfred A. Knopf, 1998), 8.

105. Ibid., 52.

106. Ibid., 297.

CHAPTER FOUR

107. Bryan Magee, *Confessions of a Philosopher* (New York: Random House, 1997), 257-8.

108. John F. Schumaker, *The Age of Insanity* (Westport, CT: Praeger Publishers, 2001). This book captures the essence of the existential anxiety of modernity.

109. Svetlana Boym, *The Future of Nostalgia* (New York: Basic Books, 2001), xiii.

110. Ibid., 17.

111. Edith Wharton, *A Backward Glance* (New York: Touchstone, 1933), xix.

112. Richard Rorty, *Philosophy and Social Hope* (New York: Penguin Books, 1999), 27. The pragmatists make the best case for creating a better world by suggesting we stop arguing over the metaphysics of injustice and instead set about fixing things.

113. Ralph Waldo Emerson, *The Portable Emerson,* ed. Carl Bode with Malcolm Cowley (New York: Penguin Books, 1946), 176-7.

114. Adam Bellow, *In Praise of Nepotism* (New York: Doubleday, 2003), 465-483. Bellow writes, "Nepotism, properly understood, is an aspect of what anthropologists call the gift economy—the system of noncommercial exchanges that serve to regulate moral relations between individuals, families, and groups in a pre-state society. This is the golden thread that links the narrow, reduced, and furtive nepotism of our time with the systematic nepotism of earlier societies going back to the first hunter-gathers. As we have seen, America is not a country without nepotism; on the contrary, it is teeming with nepotism of every kind, at every level. But because our narrow conception of nepotism as favoritism for the undeserving is still at odds with our public creed of equality and merit, America lacks a positive statement of nepotism as an ethical activity. How can nepotism be practiced in a way that does not conflict with democratic values and ideals?" How indeed? Bellow continues, "America has been called a universal nation, and it is now commonly argued that individualism is the highest good and that only by rising above our narrow and parochial connections to family, community, or ethnic group can we achieve the national unity we crave. Yet in truth, America does not invite the world to abandon the idea of kinship. Rather, America extends its inclusive vision of kinship to the world." If only we could all agree to make this effort.

115. Edward O. Wilson, *The Future of Life* (New York: Alfred A. Knopf, 2002), 23. Here Wilson tells us that if every person

on Planet Earth were to consume natural resources in the style and quantity to which we are accustomed in America, the result would require four more planets of equal size to make up the difference. Now, whether the poorest of the poor should ever reach that end is doubtful, but their aspirations to improve their lot in life are soon going to make this problem seem like a real threat to humanity at large. Their efforts will fully expose the notion of our human family in the context of a threat. But what if Wilson is exaggerating? What if he's off by 75 percent? That still leaves one planet needed, so where are we going to get it? Of course, this is only one kind of imagined threat, not to mention war, terrorism, disease, and natural catastrophe.

116. Richard Rorty, *Philosophy and Social Hope* (New York: Penguin Books, 1999), 82. Rorty says, "Moral progress is a matter of wider and wider sympathy. It is not a matter of rising above the sentimental to the rational." I suggest we think about it differently. Morality in a global sense is a case for rising above the rational to a reasonable position about the emotional bonds that we share at the family level. On page 84, Rorty says, "Once you drop the distinction between reason and passion, you no longer discriminate against a good idea because of its origins." This is my point.

117. Critics will argue that this approach is naïve, and yet it is less so than continuing to live as if we can keep relating to others as we have always done. How else can we expect to come up with results which are in any way more satisfying than the status quo?

118. Robert Wright, *The Moral Animal* (New York: Pantheon, 1994), 160. Wright says, "Brotherly love in the literal sense comes at the expense of brotherly love in the biblical sense; the more precisely we bestow unconditional kindness on relatives, the less of it is left over for others."

119. Richard Dawkins, *A Devil's Chaplin* (New York: Houghton Mifflin, 2003), 11. Dawkins writes, "If you seem to smell inconsistency or even contradiction, you are mistaken. There is no inconsistency in favoring Darwinism as an academic scientist while opposing it as a human being; any more than there is inconsistency in explaining cancer as

an academic doctor while fighting it as a practicing one."

120. Charles Darwin, *The Descent of Man* (Amherst, NY: Prometheus Books, 1998), 126-127.

121. Steven Johnson, *Emergence* (New York: Simon & Schuster, 2001), 13.

122. In her book *In a Different Voice* (Cambridge, MA: Harvard Univ. Press, 1993), Carol Gilligan takes exception to Kohlberg's Theory of Moral Development, arguing that Kohlberg's model represents a patriarchal view of life and that, from a feminist or matriarchal perspective, level three comes built-in with the nurturing aspects of motherhood and would be readily apparent but for male aggression. I'm sympathetic with this view, but the issue is a matter for others to argue. My point is that taking action to extend the notion of relating to humanity at large is more important than theories about doing so. In other words, it's the relating that matters most.

123. Robert Bly, *The Sibling Society* (New York: Vintage Books, 1996), 44.

124. John Taylor Gatto, "Against School," *Harpers*, September 2003, 33-38. Gatto argues that mandatory schooling has had the effect of making us little else but docile employees and pliable consumers.

125. Marcelo Gleiser, *The Prophet and the Astronomer* (New York: W.W. Norton, 2001), 179. Other examples of books by authors who have reached similar conclusions are Robert Wright's *Nonzero*, and Frank Tipler's *The Physics of Immortality*.

126. Aristotle was Plato's star pupil and a critic of his teacher. He concluded that Plato's abstract Forms weren't something separate from us but were within us. I think Aristotle was right about this.

127. Lou Marinoff, *Plato Not Prozac* (New York: HarperCollins, 1999).

128. Jared Diamond, *Guns, Germs, and Steel* (New York: W.W. Norton, 1997), 283.

129. Erik H. Erikson, Joan M. Erikson, and Helen Q. Kivnick, *Vital Involvement in Old Age* (New York: W.W. Norton, 1986), 36.

130. George E. Vaillant, *Aging Well* (New York: Little, Brown, 2002), 50. Vaillant adds the caveat to Erikson's life-stage

theory that one stage of life is not better or more virtuous than another. He says, "Adult development is neither a footrace nor a moral imperative. It is a road map to help us make sense of where we and where our neighbors might be located." Agreed, but for us as individuals, a failure to reach maturity is still an omission and a loss. If this were not true, then the very words maturity and development would be rendered meaningless.

131. Ibid., 45. Being a keeper of the meaning allows one to link the past with the future. On page 115, Vaillant makes the interesting observation that generativity attempted before maturity may fail in the same sense that wheat must be ripened before one can make bread.

132. Howard Gardner, Mihaly Csikszentmihalyi, and William Damon, *Good Work* (New York: Basic Books, 2001). These authors make this point repeatedly.

133. Immanuel Kant, "An Answer to the Question: 'What Is Enlightenment?'" in *Kant's Political Writings*, trans. H. B. Nisbet (Cambridge, U.K.: Cambridge Univ. Press, 1970), 54.

134. Immanuel Kant, "The Critique of Pure Reason," trans. J.M.D. Meiklejohn and W. Hastie, in *Great Books of the Western World*, Vol. 42 (Chicago: Encyclopedia Britannica, 1952), 236.

135. Ronald Gross, *Socrates' Way* (New York: Tarcher/Putnam, 2002), 29. Ronald Gross is himself a carrier of the torch and has been for many years. His *Independent Scholar's Handbook* was instrumental in helping me gain the self-confidence to take my self-education seriously.

136. Cicero, *On the Good Life,* trans. Michael Grant (New York: Penguin Books, 1971), 128.

137. Henry David Thoreau, *The Portable Thoreau*, ed. Carl Bode (New York: Penguin Books, 1947), 343-344.

138. John Holt, *Learning All the Time* (Reading, MA: Perseus Books, 1989), 128.

139. Neil Postman, *The Disappearance of Childhood* (New York: Vintage Books, 1994), 1.

BIBLIOGRAPHY

Adler, Mortimer J. *A Guidebook to Learning*. New York: Macmillan, 1986.

Allman, William F. *The Stone Age Present*. New York: Simon & Schuster, 1994.

Allport, Gordon W. *The Person in Psychology*. Boston: Beacon Press, 1968.

———. *Becoming*. New Haven, CT: Yale Univ. Press, 1955.

———. *The Nature of Prejudice*. Reading, MA: Addison-Wesley, 1954.

Anderson, Walter Truett. *The Truth About the Truth*. New York: Tarcher/Putnam, 1995.

———. *Reality Isn't What It Used To Be*. San Francisco: Harper & Row, 1990.

Arendt, Hannah. *The Life of the Mind*. New York: Harcourt, 1971.

Aristotle. "On Poetics." Translated by Ingram Bywater. In *Great Books of the Western World*. Vol. 42. Chicago: Encyclopedia Britannica, 1952.

Aurelius, Marcus. "The Meditations of Marcus Aurelius." Translated by George Long. In *Great Books of the Western World*. Vol. 12. Chicago: Encyclopedia Britannica, 1952.

Becker, Ernest. *The Denial of Death*. New York: The Free Press, 1973.

Bellow, Adam. *In Praise of Nepotism: A Natural History*. New York: Doubleday, 2003.

Bellow, Saul. *Herzog*. New York: Penguin Books, 1961.

Berman, Morris. *The Twilight of American Culture*. New York: W.W. Norton, 2000.

———. *Wandering God: A Study in Nomad Spirituality*. New York: State Univ. of New York Press, 2000.

Bloom, Harold. *How to Read and Why*. New York: Scribner, 2000.

Bly, Robert. *The Sibling Society*. New York: Vintage Books, 1996.

Boorstin, Daniel J. *The Seekers: The Story of Man's Quest to Understand His World*. New York: Random House, 1998.

———. "The Amateur Spirit." In *Living Philosophies*. Edited by Clifton Fadiman. New York: Doubleday, 1990.

Botton, Alain de. *The Consolations of Philosophy*. New York: Pantheon Books, 2000.

———. *How Proust Can Change Your Life: Not a Novel*. New York: Vintage Books, 1997.

Boym, Svetlana. *The Future of Nostalgia*. New York: Basic Books, 2001.

Campbell, Joseph. *Myths to Live By*. New York: Bantam Books, 1973.

Camus, Albert. *The Stranger*. New York: Vintage Books, 1989.

Cicero. *On the Good Life*. Translated by Michael Grant. New York: Penguin Classics, 1971.

Claxton, Guy. *Wise Up: The Challenge of Lifelong Learning*. New York: Bloomsbury Publishing, 1999.

———. *Hare Brain, Tortoise Mind: How Intelligence Increases When You Think Less*. Hopewell, NJ: Ecco Press, 1997.

Collins, Randall. *The Sociology of Philosophies: A Global Theory of Intellectual Change*. Cambridge, MA: Belknap Press of Harvard Univ. Press, 1998.

Côté, James. *Arrested Adulthood: The Changing Nature of Maturity and Identity*. New York: New York Univ. Press, 2000.

Cottom, Daniel. *Why Education Is Useless*. Philadelphia, PA: Univ. of Pennsylvania Press, 2003.

Csikszentmihalyi, Mihaly. *Creativity: Flow and the Psychology of Discovery and Invention*. New York: HarperCollins, 1996.

———. *The Evolving Self: A Psychology for the Third Millennium*. New York: HarperCollins, 1993.

———. *Flow: The Psychology of Optimal Experience*. New York: Harper & Row, 1990.

Dalai Lama XIV. *The Power of Compassion*. San Francisco: Thorsons, 1995.

Darwin, Charles. *The Descent of Man*. Amherst, NY: Prometheus Books, 1998.

Davidson, Richard J., and Anne Harrington. *Visions of Compassion: Western Scientists and Tibetan Buddhists*

Examine Human Nature. New York: Oxford Univ. Press, 2002.

Dawkins, Richard. *A Devil's Chaplin: Reflections on Hope, Lies, Science and Love.* New York: Houghton Mifflin, 2003.

Deci, Edward L., and Richard Flaste. *Why We Do What We Do: Understanding Self-Motivation.* New York: Penguin Books, 1995.

Dennett, Daniel C. *Freedom Evolves.* New York: Viking Press, 2003.

———. *Darwin's Dangerous Idea.* New York: Simon & Schuster, 1995.

Diamond, Jared. *Guns, Germs, and Steel: The Fates of Human Societies.* New York: W.W. Norton, 1997.

Dobson, Linda. *What the Rest of Us Can Learn from Homeschooling.* New York: Three Rivers Press, 2003.

Dychtwald, Ken. *Age Power: How the 21st Century Will Be Ruled by the New Old.* Los Angeles, CA: Tarcher/Putnam, 1999.

———. *Age Wave: How the Most Important Trend of Our Time Will Change Our Future.* Los Angeles, CA: Jeremy P. Tarcher, 1989.

Ellison, Ralph. *Invisible Man.* New York: Vintage Books, 1995.

Emerson, Ralph Waldo. *Emerson Essays and Lectures.* New York: The Library of America, 1983.

———. *The Portable Emerson.* Edited by Carl Bode with Malcolm Cowley. New York: Penguin Books, 1946.

Enright, D.J., ed. *The Oxford Book of Death.* New York: Oxford Univ. Press, 1983.

Epictetus. *The Art of Living.* Interpreted by Sharon Lebell. New York: HarperCollins, 1994.

Erikson, Erik H. *Identity and the Life Cycle.* New York: W.W. Norton, 1980.

Erikson, Erik H., Joan M. Erikson, and Helen Q. Kivnick. *Vital Involvement in Old Age.* New York: W.W. Norton, 1986.

Evans, Dylan. *Emotion: The Science of Sentiment.* New York: Oxford Univ. Press, 2001.

Festinger, Leon. *A Theory of Cognitive Dissonance.* Stanford, CA: Stanford Univ. Press, 1962.

Feyerabend, Paul. *Conquest of Abundance: A Tale of Abstraction Versus the Richness of Being.* Chicago: Univ. of Chicago Press, 1999.

Fisher, James R., Jr., *In the Shadow of the Courthouse.*

Bloomington, IN: 1stBooks, 2003.

Flanagan, Owen. *The Problem of the Soul: Two Visions of the Mind and How to Reconcile Them.* New York: Basic Books, 2002.

Frank, Robert H. *Luxury Fever.* New York: The Free Press, 1999.

Frankl, Viktor. *Man's Search for Meaning.* New York: Pocket Books, 1984.

Fromm, Erich. *The Sane Society.* New York: Rinehart & Winston, 1955.

Gandhi, Mohandas K. *The Words of Gandhi.* Selected by Richard Attenborough. New York: New Market Press, 1982.

Gardner, Howard. *The Disciplined Mind: What All Students Should Understand.* New York: Simon & Schuster, 1999.

———. *Frames of Mind: The Theory of Multiple Intelligences.* New York: Basic Books, 1993.

Gardner, Howard, Mihaly Csikszentmihalyi, and William Damon. *Good Work: When Excellence and Ethics Meet.* New York: Basic Books, 2001.

Gatto, John Taylor. "Against School." *Harpers*, September 2003, 33-38.

———. *Dumbing Us Down: The Hidden Curriculum of Compulsory Schooling.* Gabriola Island, BC: New Society Publishers, 1992.

Geldard, Richard. *The Spiritual Teachings of Ralph Waldo Emerson.* Great Barrington, MA: Lindisfarne Books, 2001.

Gibbs, John C. *Moral Development and Reality: Beyond the Theories of Kohlberg and Hoffman.* Thousand Oaks, CA: Sage Publications, 2003.

Gilligan, Carol. *In a Different Voice: Psychological Theory and Women's Development.* Cambridge, MA: Harvard Univ. Press, 1993.

Glassner, Barry. *The Culture of Fear: Why Americans Are Afraid of the Wrong Things.* New York: Basic Books, 1999.

Gleiser, Marcelo. *The Prophet and the Astronomer: A Scientific Journey to the End of Time.* New York: W.W. Norton, 2001.

Goldstein, Joseph. *One Dharma: The Emerging Western Buddhism.* New York: HarperCollins, 2002.

Graber, Robert Bates. *Valuing Useless Knowledge.* Kirksville, MO: Thomas Jefferson Univ. Press, 1995.

Graff, Gerald. *Clueless in Academe: How Schooling Obscures the Life of the Mind.* New Haven, CT: Yale Univ. Press, 2003.

Grant, George. *Time as History*. Toronto, ON: University of Toronto Press, 1995.

Greider, William. *The Soul of Capitalism: Opening Paths to a Moral Economy*. New York: Simon & Schuster, 2003.

———. *One World, Ready or Not: The Manic Logic of Global Capitalism*. New York: Simon & Schuster, 1997.

Griffin, Joe, and Ivan Tyrrell. *Human Givens: A New Approach to Emotional Health and Clear Thinking*. Chalvington, East Sussex, United Kingdom: Human Givens Publishing, 2003.

Gross, Ronald. *Socrates' Way: Seven Master Keys to Using Your Mind to the Utmost*. New York: Jeremy P. Tarcher/Putnam, 2002.

———. The *Independent Scholar's Handbook*. Berkeley, CA: Ten Speed Press, 1993.

———. *Peak Learning: How to Create Your Own Lifelong Education Program for Personal Enlightenment and Professional Success*. New York: Jeremy P. Tarcher/ Putnam, 1991.

Hayes, Charles D. *Portals in a Northern Sky*. Wasilla, AK: Autodidactic Press, 2003.

———. *Training Yourself: The Twenty-First Century Credential*. Wasilla, AK: Autodidactic Press, 2000.

———. *Beyond the American Dream: Lifelong Learning and the Search for Meaning in a Postmodern World*. Wasilla, AK: Autodidactic Press, 1998.

———. *Proving You're Qualified: Strategies for Competent People without College Degrees*. Wasilla, AK: Autodidactic Press, 1995.

———. *Self-University: The Price of Tuition is the Desire to Learn. Your Degree is a Better Life*. Wasilla, AK: Autodidactic Press, 1989.

Heilbrun, Carolyn G. *The Last Gift of Time: Life Beyond Sixty*. New York: Ballantine Books, 1997.

Hemingway, Ernest. *A Farewell to Arms*. New York: Scribner, 1929.

Hillman, James. *The Force of Character: And the Lasting Life*. New York: Random House, 1999.

Hirth, Diane. "Wiesel Warns of Indifference." Fort Lauderdale *Sun Sentinel*, May 8, 1987.

Hoffer, Eric. *The True Believer: Thoughts on the Nature of Mass Movements*. New York: Harper & Row, 1951.

Hofstadter, Richard. *Anti-Intellectualism in American Life*. New York: Vintage Books, 1962.

Holt, John. *Learning All the Time*. Reading, MA: Perseus Books, 1989.

Hudson, Frederic M. *The Adult Years: Mastering the Art of Self-Renewal*. San Francisco: Jossey-Bass, 1999.

Hume, David. *A Treatise of Human Nature*. Edited by L.A. Selby-Bigge. London: Oxford at the Clarendon Press, 1888.

Inghilleri, Paolo. *From Subjective Experience to Cultural Change*. Translated by Eleonora Bartoli. New York: Cambridge Univ. Press, 1999.

Jacobson, David. *Emerson's Pragmatic Vision: The Dance of the Eye*. Univ. Park, PA: Pennsylvania State Univ. Press, 1993.

Johnson, Steven. *Emergence: The Connected Lives of Ants, Brains, Cities, and Software*. New York: Simon & Schuster, 2001.

Kant Immanuel. "An Answer to the Question: 'What Is Enlightenment?'" Translated by H. B. Nisbet. In *Kant's Political Writings*. Cambridge, U.K.: Cambridge Univ. Press, 1970.

———. "The Critique of Pure Reason," "The Critique of Practical Reason," and "The Metaphysic of Morals." Translated by J. M. D. Meiklejohn and W. Hastie. In *Great Books of the Western World*. Vol. 42. Chicago: Encyclopedia Britannica, 1952.

Kegan, Robert. *In Over Our Heads: The Mental Demands of Modern Life*. Cambridge, MA: Harvard Univ. Press, 1994.

Kierkegaard, Søren. *The Sickness Unto Death*. Edited and translated by Howard V. Hong and Edna H. Hong. Princeton, NJ: Princeton Univ. Press, 1980.

Knowles, Malcolm S. *The Adult Learner: A Neglected Species*. Houston: Gulf Publishing, 1990.

———. *The Modern Practice of Adult Education: From Pedagogy to Andragogy*. Chicago: Follett, 1980.

Kohlberg, Lawrence. *The Psychology of Moral Development*. San Francisco: Harper & Row, 1984.

Kundera, Milan. *Ignorance*. New York: HarperCollins, 2000.

Kushner, Harold S. *Living a Life That Matters*. New York: Alfred A. Knopf, 2001.

Lakoff, George, and Mark Johnson. *Philosophy in the Flesh: The Embodied Mind and Its Challenge to Western Thought.* New York: Basic Books, 1999.

———. *Metaphors We Live By.* Chicago: Univ. of Chicago Press, 1980.

Landman, Janet. *Regret: The Persistence of the Possible.* New York: Oxford Univ. Press, 1993.

Langer, Ellen J. *Mindfulness.* New York: Addison-Wesley, 1989.

Levine, Mel. *A Mind at a Time: America's Top Learning Expert Shows How Every Child Can Succeed.* New York: Simon & Schuster, 2002.

Magee, Bryan. *Confessions of a Philosopher: A Personal Journey Through Western Philosophy from Plato to Popper.* New York: Random House, 1997.

———. *The Philosophy of Schopenhauer.* New York: Oxford Univ. Press, 1983.

Marinoff, Lou. *Plato Not Prozac: Applying Eternal Wisdom to Everyday Problems.* New York: HarperCollins, 1999.

Markos, Louis. *From Plato to Postmodernism: Understanding the Essence of Literature and the Role of the Author.* Kearneysville, WV: The Teaching Company, 1999. Audiocassette.

Maslow, Abraham H. *The Farther Reaches of Human Nature.* New York: Viking Press, 1971.

McEwan, Ian. *Atonement.* New York: First Anchor Books, 2003.

Miller, Matthew. *The 2 Percent Solution: Fixing America's Problems in Ways Liberals and Conservatives Can Love.* New York: Public Affairs, 2003.

Morrow, Lance. *Evil: An Investigation.* New York: Basic Books, 2003.

Murdoch, Iris. *Metaphysics as a Guide to Morals.* New York: Viking Penguin, 1992.

Nehamas, Alexander. *The Art of Living: Socratic Reflections from Plato to Foucault.* Berkeley, CA: Univ. of California Press, 1998.

Neiman, Susan. *Evil in Modern Thought: An Alternative History of Philosophy.* Princeton, NJ: Princeton Univ. Press, 2002.

Nietzsche, Friedrich. *The Portable Nietzsche.* Edited and translated by Walter Kaufmann. New York: Penguin Books, 1982.

————. *Beyond Good and Evil.* Edited and translated by R. J. Hollindale. New York: Penguin Books, 1973.

Nussbaum, Martha Craven. *Cultivating Humanity.* Cambridge, MA: Harvard Univ. Press, 1998.

Nuttall, A.D. *Why Does Tragedy Give Pleasure?* New York: Oxford Univ. Press, 1996.

O'Toole, Patricia. *Money and Morals in America.* New York: Clarkson Potter, 1998.

Owen, David. *Maturity and Modernity: Nietzsche, Weber, Foucault and the Ambivalence of Reason.* London: Rutledge, 1994.

Parfit, Derek. *Reasons and Persons.* New York: Oxford Univ. Press, 1984.

Peck, M. Scott. *Further Along the Road Less Traveled: The Unending Journey Toward Spiritual Growth.* New York: Touchstone Books, 1998.

————. *The Road Less Traveled.* New York: Simon & Schuster, 1978.

Pinker, Steven. *The Blank Slate: The Modern Denial of Human Nature.* New York: Viking, 2002.

————. *How the Mind Works.* New York: W.W. Norton, 1997.

Pipes, Daniel. *Conspiracy: How the Paranoid Style Flourishes and Where It Comes From.* New York: Touchstone Books, 1999.

Pipher, Mary. *Another Country: Navigating the Emotional Terrain of Our Elders.* New York: Riverhead Books, 1999.

Plato. "The Dialogues of Plato." Translated by Benjamin Jowett. In *Great Books of the Western World.* Vol. 7. Chicago: Encyclopedia Britannica, 1952.

Postman, Neil. *Building a Bridge to the Eighteenth Century.* New York: Alfred A. Knopf, 1999.

————. *The Disappearance of Childhood.* New York: Vintage Books, 1994.

————. *Amusing Ourselves to Death.* New York: Viking Penguin, 1985.

Postrel, Virginia. *The Substance of Style: How the Rise of Aesthetic Value is Remaking Commerce, Culture, and Consciousness.* New York: HarperCollins, 2003.

Power, Samantha. *A Problem from Hell: America and the Age of Genocide.* New York: Basic Books, 2002.

Rawls, John. *A Theory of Justice.* Cambridge, MA: Belknap

Press of Harvard Univ. Press, 1971.

Richardson, Robert D., Jr., *Emerson: The Mind on Fire*. Berkeley, CA: Univ. of California Press, 1995.

Riesman, David. *The Lonely Crowd*. New Haven, CT: Yale Univ. Press, 2001.

Roderick, Rick. *The Self Under Siege*. Kearneysville, WV: The Teaching Company, 1993. Audiocassette.

————. *Philosophy and Human Values*. Kearneysville, WV: The Teaching Company, 1991. Audiocassette.

Rorty, Richard. *Philosophy and Social Hope*. New York: Penguin Books, 1999.

Roszak, Theodore. *America the Wise: The Longevity Revolution and the Real Wealth of Nations*. New York: Houghton Mifflin, 1998.

Sagan, Carl. *Contact*. New York: Doubleday, 1997.

————. *The Demon-Haunted World: Science as a Candle in the Dark*. New York: Ballantine Books, 1997.

Samples, Bob. *The Metaphoric Mind: A Celebration of Creative Consciousness*. Reading, MA: Addison-Wesley, 1976.

Santayana, George. *Skepticism and Animal Faith*. New York: Dover, 1923.

Sartre, Jean Paul. *Being and Nothingness: A Phenomenological Essay on Ontology*. Translated by Hazel E. Barnes. New York: Washington Square Press, 1993.

Schacht, Richard. *Making Sense of Nietzsche*. Chicago: Univ. of Illinois Press, 1995.

Schmidt, Jeff. *Disciplined Minds: A Critical Look at Salaried Professionals and the Soul-Battering System that Shapes Their Lives*. Lanham, MD: Rowman & Littlefield, 2000.

Schopenhauer, Arthur. *Studies in Pessimism*. Translated by T. Bailey Saunders. London: George Allen & Company, 1913.

Schumaker, John F. *The Age of Insanity: Modernity and Mental Health*. Westport, CT: Praeger, 2001.

Seneca. *Seneca: Letters from a Stoic*. Edited and translated by Robin Campbell. New York: Penguin Books, 1969.

Sennett, Richard. *Respect in a World of Inequality*. New York: W.W. Norton, 2003.

Shaw, George Bernard. *Man and Superman*. New York: Brentano's, 1903.

Shermer, Michael. *Why People Believe Weird Things: Pseudoscience,*

Superstition, and Other Confusions of Our Time. New York: W. H. Freeman, 1998.

Singer, Peter. *How Are We to Live?* New York: Prometheus Books, 1995.

Slater, Philip E. *A Dream Deferred: America's Discontent and Search for a New Democratic Ideal*. Boston, MA: Beacon Press, 1991.

———. *The Pursuit of Loneliness*, 3rd ed. Boston, MA: Beacon Press, 1990.

Smith, Harmon. *My Friend, My Friend: The Story of Thoreau's Relationship with Emerson*. Amherst, MA: Univ. of Massachusetts Press, 1999.

Smoot, George, and Keay Davidson. *Wrinkles in Time*. London: Little, Brown, 1993.

Solomon, Robert C. *Spirituality for the Skeptic*. New York, NY: Oxford Univ. Press, 2002.

———. *A Passion for Justice*. New York: Addison-Wesley, 1990.

Stack, George J. *Nietzsche and Emerson*. Athens, OH: Ohio Univ. Press, 1992.

Staub, Ervin. *The Psychology of Good and Evil: Why Children, Adults, and Groups Help and Harm Others*. New York: Cambridge Univ. Press, 2003.

Sternberg, Robert J., and Todd I. Lubart. *Defying the Crowd: Cultivating Creativity in a Culture of Conformity*. New York: The Free Press, 1995.

Taylor, Shelley E. *Positive Illusions*. New York: Basic Books, 1989.

Thoreau, Henry David. *The Portable Thoreau*. Edited by Carl Bode. New York: Penguin Books, 1947.

Tipler, Frank J. *The Physics of Immortality: Modern Cosmology, God and the Resurrection of the Dead*. New York: Anchor Books, 1997.

Turiel, Elliot. *The Culture of Morality: Social Development, Context, and Conflict*. New York: Cambridge Univ. Press, 2002.

Twitchell, James B. *Living It Up: America's Love Affair with Luxury*. New York: Columbia Univ. Press, 2002.

Vaillant, George E. *Aging Well: Surprising Guideposts to a Happier Life from the Landmark Harvard Study of Adult Development*. New York: Little, Brown, 2002.

Watts, Alan. *The Wisdom of Insecurity*. New York: Vintage Books, 1951.

Waugh, Alexander. *Time: Its Origin, Its Enigma, Its History*. New York: Carroll & Graf, 1999.

Weinberg, Steven. *Facing Up: Science and Its Cultural Adversaries*. Cambridge, MA: Harvard Univ. Press, 2001

Wharton, Edith. *A Backward Glance*. New York: Touchstone, 1933.

Wilson, Edward O. *The Future of Life*. New York: Alfred A. Knopf, 2002.

————. *Consilience: The Unity of Knowledge*. New York: Alfred A. Knopf, 1998.

————. *The Diversity of Life*. Cambridge, MA: Belknap Press of Harvard Univ. Press, 1992.

Woodruff, Paul. *Reverence: Renewing a Forgotten Virtue*. New York: Oxford Univ. Press, 2001.

Wright, Robert. *Nonzero: The Logic of Human Destiny*. New York: Vintage Books, 2001.

————. *The Moral Animal: Why We Are the Way We Are: The New Science of Evolutionary Psychology*. New York: Pantheon Books, 1994.

INDEX

ABOUT THE AUTHOR

A uthor and publisher Charles D. Hayes is a self-taught philosopher and one of America's strongest advocates for lifelong learning. He spent his youth in Texas and served as a U.S. Marine and a police officer before embarking on a career in the oil industry. Alaska has been his home for more than 25 years.

Hayes' book *Beyond the American Dream: Lifelong Learning and the Search for Meaning in a Postmodern World* received recognition by the American Library Association's *CHOICE* Magazine as one of the most outstanding academic books of the year. His other titles include *Training Yourself: The 21st Century Credential; Proving You're Qualified: Strategies for Competent People without College Degrees;* and *Self-University: The Price of Tuition is Desire. Your Degree is a Better Life.* In 2003, he published his first novel, *Portals in a Northern Sky.*

Promoting the idea that education should be thought of not as something you get but as something you take, Hayes' work has been featured in *USA Today*, in the *UTNE Reader*, and on National Public Radio's *Talk of the Nation.* His web site, www.autodidactic.com, provides resources for self-directed learners—from advice about credentials to philosophy about the value lifelong learning brings to everyday living.

ALSO BY CHARLES D. HAYES

Portals in a Northern Sky

Training Yourself: The 21ˢᵗ Century Credential

Beyond the American Dream: Lifelong Learning and the Search for Meaning in a Postmodern World

Proving You're Qualified: Strategies for Competent People without College Degrees

Self-University: The Price of Tuition is the Desire to Learn. Your Degree is a Better Life